VACCINATIONS
THE REST OF THE STORY

Most of the articles, letters, and reviews in this book appeared originally in Mothering *magazine between 1979–1992.*

Published by Mothering, *PO Box 1690, Santa Fe, NM 87504.*
Printed in the United States of America.
Printed on recycled paper.

Editor: Peggy O'Mara
Project Editor: Carol Newfeld
Copyeditor: Ann Mason
Designer: Mary Shapiro
Cover Photo: Suzanne Arms

ISBN 0-914257-10-2

VACCINATIONS
THE REST OF THE STORY

*A Selection of Articles, Letters, and Resources
1979-1992*

MOTHERING SPECIAL EDITION

CONTENTS

BOOK REVIEWS

Immunizations: Risks and Rates

YOUR CHOICE

Nineteen years ago, when I was pregnant with my first child, I began to ask questions about vaccinations. The reactions to these questions were so vehement that I realized I was considered a social deviant for even questioning what others took for granted. It was nearly impossible to find answers. Those in favor of vaccinations considered my questions so irresponsible that they wouldn't bother to engage in debate. Those opposed were so sensational in their arguments that I was left unsatisfied.

My answers came primarily from my own experience. A biologist told me that there were some valid immunological concerns about vaccinations. La Leche League referred me to consulting physicians who cautiously suggested that it might be acceptable to delay vaccinations. In the end, it was the mother in me who won out. I simply could never take my well baby in to be made sick. This "just in case" reasoning behind vaccinations continues to befuddle me.

I have four children ranging in age from 10 to 18. Not one has been vaccinated. We have survived measles, chicken pox, pneumonia, and meningitis, as well as medical emergencies of other sorts. I am not self-righteous enough to believe that my alternative views on health, my diet, or my good karma have protected my family from the ravages of disease that vaccine proponents fear. However, I do believe that my children have stronger immune systems than they would have had if they had been vaccinated. I have never regretted my decision not to vaccinate them.

On the other hand, I am not an antivaccine proselytizer; nor do I stand on a soapbox. I made a decision for my family. I have no investment in what others do except to provide solid information on which to base informed choice. Whatever family health decisions we make, I know we feel better in the future when they are informed, personal, and well thought out. If we do what others think is right without finding out if it is right for us, we risk regrets in later life.

The mandating of vaccines is of greatest concern to me. While vaccines are compulsory, we have no real information about their pros and cons. There are too many vested interests in them to know what is true. Health care in the United States has become so standardized that we have forgotten that true science requires not automatically using a procedure or practice because it is available, but rather determining under which circumstances that procedure or practice is right for us.

Families with a history of allergies or allergic reactions to vaccines have different questions to ask themselves than families whose ancestors have been crippled by polio. We all bring our histories and our fears to the decision-making table, and we do our best when we respect the whole plate rather than blind ourselves to part of it.

I can encourage those of you who wonder how unvaccinated children turn out. I cannot tell you what is best for you. We present you here with material that we have gathered for nearly 15 years from physicians, healthcare professionals, and parents. We present resources for further study. This information is responsible and reputable in an age when AIDS has raised new questions about the nature of the immune system. We live in a world that taxes the immune system in ways we do not yet fully understand.

How best to protect and enliven the immune system is the underlying question. Much goes unanswered. Vaccines do not guarantee immunity. Forgoing vaccines does not guarantee safety. Although society leads us to believe we can control life, this is not true. Life is risky no matter how you toss the coin. And when you are responsible for others' lives, the weight of the decision making may suggest a cautious course.

Remember, you will still be in your child's life 20 years from now. Advice givers of the present may not be. You and your family are the only ones who must live with your decisions. Trust in yourself is the key. Make your decision with as much information as you can garner, then trust your intuition and take a leap of faith. Whatever your decision may be, make it one you will feel comfortable explaining to your child 20 years from now.

Peggy O'Mara
Editor/Publisher
Mothering

A MOTHER'S RESEARCH ON IMMUNIZATION

Patricia Savage

Patricia Savage lives in New Hampshire with her five children. She is a freelance writer, homeschooler, baker for a natural foods café, and self-described lover of life. An earlier version of "A Mother's Research on Immunization" first appeared in Mothering, no. 13 (Fall 1979).

Socrates said that the unexamined life was not worth living. John Holt talks about children being at a tremendous advantage as creative thinkers because they explore the world not knowing what the "right" questions are to ask—they ask them all! Both the sage and the child inspire me in this endeavor: I ask questions that do not have obvious answers. Indeed, the more questions I ask, the more questions seem to surface.

The subject is immunizations. I write not as a professional with a point of view to defend, but rather as a mother with concern about a practice that may not be in the best interest of my children's health. This article does not give any final answers to the complex question of immunization, although the reasoning that supports my feelings should help to clarify the reader's feelings. However, it does represent some refinements of the questions that I have been asking for nearly two years. If it provides access to information about immunization, then it will have fulfilled at least one objective. I encourage you to check out all of the listed references.

Another objective of this article is to support parents in their need to express their hesitations about specific medical procedures with their doctors. Professionals should ideally be seen as experts in their particular fields, able to offer valuable recommendations based on their (always limited) understanding. We as parents must make the decisions that will affect our children. No one knows all there is to know about the human body; perhaps we know $\frac{1}{1000}$ of how it functions. Therefore, our reservations about using unnatural intervention in any healthcare situation should be as respected as our consent.

A final objective is to encourage research or, more accurately, to inspire a change in the focus of research from disease-oriented to prevention-oriented. Very simply, the approach based on the search for cures is not working for many of our most common diseases. We do not have answers to cancer or diabetes or the common cold. But those are topics for other papers. Let us turn to the question: Do immunizations work?

Smallpox, diphtheria, whooping cough, and polio have now nearly been eradicated in the United States. The initial questions that crop up go something like this: What has been the effectiveness of immunization programs? Is the radical decrease in the number of persons suffering from dread disease due to inoculation programs, or are there other factors operating to keep the population free from epidemics? Do the premises that the germ theory of disease is based on stand up under modern inquiry?

Historically, medical scientists have always asked with regard to epidemics: What causes so many to become afflicted? The appeal of the germ theory of disease as an answer is in the fact that bacteria are always present upon examining diseased tissue. Pasteur's work provided an important impetus to changing the way we view personal hygiene, but the logic of bacteria as the pathogens does not hold up under more recent investigation. Bacteria of all kinds are endemic: their role is to convert decaying tissue into new healthy usable matter. These microorganisms are a product rather than a cause of disease, according to many bacteriologists. It is rare that a species will transgress the border of biologic normalcy to pathenogenicity. For this reason, some feel that the germ theory does disservice to our understanding of the true nature of disease. The idea that germs are enemies that should be destroyed or outwitted is one with which many people feel uncomfortable.

Just as good a question for scientists to ask regarding "contagious" disease might be: What causes some persons to resist disease when exposed? Any epidemic has its limits. One out of ten may be affected. Often the afflicted and the nonafflicted live in the same household. Bacteriologist Dr. Lumiere, writing in the *Revue Generale des Sciences Pures et Appliques,* has reported tubercle bacillus in the discharge and blood of persons free of tuberculosis. Interestingly enough, cultures taken from TB patients have often revealed no tubercle bacillus. Here is an example where no connection can be made between the germ and the disease. Moreover, there is the case publicized by Dr. Friederich Löffler where diphtheria bacillus could be found in the throat cultures of healthy children.

Leonard Jacobs, writing for the *East West Journal,* reports that even Pasteur was aware that fermentation (which he studied extensively while formulating his germ theory) only occurs in injured, bruised, or dead material, and that bacteria are a natural result of fermentation, not the cause.

Because of such gaps in the germ theory, it becomes important to consider what other factors could be involved in susceptibility to disease. According to researcher Eleanor McBean in her 1974 book *The Poisoned Needle,* the most noticeable decrease in smallpox occurred at the beginning of the nineteenth century with improvements in sanitation and nutrition. Sanitation reform included such things as improved housing, better water supplies, improved sewage disposal, and better transportation for carrying perishable foods to the city. Nutritional awareness was enhanced to the extent that foods were kept free from contamination through spoilage.

Other types of nutritional reform in the latter part of the century were to operate against the attainment of true health, however. When the correlation between disease and contamination of food was drawn, perhaps impetus was given to develop procedures that could further retard spoilage. Enter the refined foods industry. Removing the germ from grains such as wheat made them less likely to go rancid; pasteurizing milk reduced the rate at which bacteria could multiply; and unfertilized eggs seemed to store better. But these measures reduced the nutritional value of foods enormously. The body was being called upon to process foods deficient in the very vitamins and minerals that were needed for digestion and assimilation. A drain on the reserves of vital elements was being set up, leaving the body less able to withstand disease. I see a relationship between the diseases such as smallpox, typhoid fever, or diphtheria and sanitation problems; there also seems to be a link between devitalized foodstuffs prepared for long shelf life and the problems that plague us today: diabetes, allergy, flu, heart disease, and cancer to mention a few.

Discussion of susceptibility to disease and immunization invariably brings up the subject of antibodies, a subject that invites closer examination. Dr. Herbert M. Shelton, author of *The Hygienic System*, brings three big problems into focus:

1) Because the hypothetical substance (antibodies) cannot be isolated, injections of foreign proteins into the bloodstream are necessary. A tremendous burden may be placed on the body to deal with this foreign substance. For example, theories

attempting to explain allergy often suggest foreign proteins in the blood as possible causal agents. It should be remembered that in this country, very young babies, at a particularly vulnerable stage for development of allergy, are the ones most commonly inoculated. Also, it is interesting in this regard to consider how common it is for the baby to have symptoms of illness (fever, rash, diarrhea) in reaction to vaccination. A last point related to this consideration: Jonas Salk, creator of the polio vaccine used so extensively in the 1950s, recently testified that all the polio cases occurring since 1970 in the United States seem to have been produced by "live" polio vaccine. This is a man whose life and reputation are closely linked with vaccination, and he has raised questions about the injection of live virus into the bloodstream.

2) If antibodies fight off disease, there is still no proof that they remain in the bloodstream after the need for them ceases. The repetition of the booster shot (immunization for diphtheria, pertussis, and tetanus—DPT) is always stressed by physicians. Unfortunately, as time goes on there is a reported need for more shots (consider now that we immunize for rubella and are currently having an epidemic of rubella) and at shorter intervals (it is commonly advised that a child have up to five DPT shots by the time he or she reaches school age). It seems possible that there is some growing awareness that immunizations have their shortcomings, but rather than challenge the basic assumptions on which they are based, the medical profession deduces that better protection will be afforded through more of the same. (It seems to be necessary, according to this kind of logic, to keep the vaccine ever-present in order to keep the antibodies ever-

present. Does that bother anyone else?)

What does the record say concerning the effectiveness of immunizations? Untangling the web of statistics is difficult. The task is to find statistics that give meaningful answers. Mentioned earlier was the fact that environmental improvements brought a decline in certain diseases. It is interesting that from 1860 to 1948 in England there were dramatic decreases in measles (94.1 percent), scarlet fever (99.7 percent), and whooping cough (91 percent) without vaccinations. Diphtheria, for which serum immunization was used, decreased less significantly than these other diseases. The most dramatic decrease in incidence of diphtheria can be seen in the case of four million children who were not immunized from 1945 to 1949.

English history provides interesting facts regarding smallpox. The incidence of smallpox actually increased with the introduction of smallpox vaccine. Prior to 1853 (and the complete vaccination of the nation), there had been about 2,000 deaths per two-year period. Nearly 20 years later after the vaccination program had been in effect for those years, the biggest smallpox epidemic of 23,062 occurred. Towns where there had been the most thorough enforcement (such as Leicester, Sheffield) were the most severely hit. By 1900, the effects of health-care improvements had been weighed against the effects of inoculation, and the English began to resist immunization programs. Although the enforcement of immunization laws became lax in England, the government still managed to rigidly enforce compulsory vaccination in India. India's smallpox death rate compared very unfavorably with England's at the turn of this century. For example: Bombay, 866 deaths; Calcutta, 1,201 deaths; London, 23 deaths per million. In 1929, the League of Nations reported that India (still under Britain) was "the greatest center of smallpox today."

In our country, smallpox vaccination lost its appeal about 1927 when it was realized that the vaccinated suffered the worst effects of the disease. A brief look at the statistics for the United States reveals the following: In 1902, there were 2,121 deaths from smallpox, when use of the smallpox vaccine was at its height; by 1927, there were 138, when it had for the most part been abandoned. Around this time there was a ten-year campaign of vaccination against smallpox in the Philippines; the death rate rose from 10 percent to 74 percent. In 1918, more than 18,000 Filipinos died from smallpox. As late as the 1950s, countries such as Mexico, where little improvement in sanitation has been made over the years—particularly sewage disposal—smallpox was still very much a problem. Compulsory vaccination had not been any more of an answer in that country than it had been elsewhere.

These facts do not make a good case for the effectiveness of the smallpox vaccine. The case is similar for polio if one looks at those statistics. The statistics quoted for smallpox, as well as those for polio, can be found in *The Poisoned Needle.* They are worth your time.

In addition to the questionable effectiveness of vaccines, my investigation brought up another profoundly disturbing question: What are the risks of serious side effects? Dr. Robert Mendelsohn has published some interesting observations in his newsletter *The People's Doctor.* For example, the risk of death from smallpox vaccine is now greater than the risk of death from smallpox itself. An acquaintance was planning a trip to South America and was required to have both herself and her one year old vaccinated for smallpox. Ten days later the baby had, she was told, spinal meningitis from which he almost died. Dr. Mendelsohn quotes Dr. Robert Simpson speaking at a seminar of the American Cancer Society: ". . . immunization programs against flu, measles, mumps, polio, etc., actually may be seeding humans with RNA to form proviruses which will then become latent cells throughout the body. Some of these latent proviruses could be molecules in search of diseases which under proper conditions become activated and cause a variety of diseases, including rheumatoid arthritis, multiple sclerosis, lupus erythematosus, Parkinson's disease and perhaps cancer."

The medical profession admits that there are possible complications arising from the use of any vaccine. But often the family pediatrician relates this to the patient by saying that the risks are hardly considerable compared to the risks of the disease itself. This is misleading—actually in many instances it is false. There are many side effects from smallpox vaccine (encephalitis, eczema vaccinatum, accidental implant of vaccinia on the eye, superinfection of other skin conditions). The side effects for whooping cough vaccine include high fever, convulsions, and encephalopathy, while those for measles include encephalitis, subacute sclerosing panencephalitis, ataxia, retardation, learning disability, hyperactivity, aseptic meningitis, seizure disorders, and hemiparesis. These are the more commonly seen complications as described by the medical profession. I worry about the extent of side effects not yet questioned by doctors resulting from vaccination. No one can offer guarantees that your child will not become more susceptible to ear infection, or colds, or skin rash as a result of this procedure. (My son's only illness the first year of life was an ear infection that he got two weeks after a DPT shot.) Simply because the physician has not made a connection between those symptoms and inoculation does not assure us that none exists. Assurances cannot be made, and if they are—beware.

Other interesting facts with regard to assurances are the following: 1) Today, parents of schoolchildren sign a paper agreeing not to sue if complications arise from compulsory immunizations. 2) In California, there is a new law providing up to $25,000 for medical expenses for children who have *catastrophic* reactions to mandatory immunizations. In the words of Marian Tompson, "The fact that this law was enacted makes me feel that such reactions can't be all that rare!" Somehow reading this, the ghastly pictures in *The Poisoned Needle* seem more believable and the author's slightly hysterical tone more understandable. In our town, the school has requested that the students update their inoculations with a new measles shot before entering high school. There have been several recent epidemics of measles in our area, primarily affecting teens. Not only are their bouts with this illness more severe, they also are at greater risk than younger children for long-term consequences.

With such developments that undermine the theory of inoculation, the ultimate question becomes: If immunization does not ensure good health, what does?

Being discontent with superficial answers, I first had to ask myself: What is health? What is disease? I accept the definition of health as 100 percent of the body functioning 100 percent normally 100 percent of the time. Disease is an interruption of that ideal state. Symptoms of disease are an indication that the body is using extraordinary measures to eliminate excess waste or toxins. For example, mucus discharge, diarrhea, vomiting, fever, skin rash, and so forth can be signs that the normal channels of detoxification (such as through the liver) are overloaded and new outlets are being sought for elimination. Germs feed on toxic waste matter, so it becomes important to know what kinds of things can cause toxicity. Or what kinds of things can be done to prevent disease.

As in all things, there is not just one answer. The observation that I am able to make after considerable investigation is that there seem to be four things that form a common thread running through all health philosophies: 1) diet, 2) exercise, 3) relaxation, and 4) positive attitude. In addition, I would add 5) making use of the many alternative preventative healthcare systems, such as acupuncture, homeopathy, chiropractic, herbology, therapeutic massage, and reflexology.

Diet. Discussions on diet are always controversial but still worth engaging in. Along with Henry Bieler and Maxine Block, authors of *Food Is Your Best Medicine,* I feel that proper diet is the best protection against disease. Breastfeeding is the ideal: in addition to the emotional benefits both to the baby and mother, the nutritional advantages cannot be stressed enough. The newborn who is provided with the initial colostrum as well as the subsequent milk is getting exactly what nature has designed for his or her body. All the vitamins that are present will be available to the baby; that is, there is no loss due to processing or heating as in the case of formula. Moreover, immunological factors have been isolated by scientists. Mother's milk contains immunoglobulins, assigned names such as secretory IgA, IgG, IgM, and so forth. IgA works to bind viruses and bacteria in the stomach, preventing them from invading the mucosa. One of the unique properties of this substance is that it resists stomach enzymes, which guarantees its survival. To me, that is a better assurance than using vaccines whose stability in the bloodstream may be questionable.

Once solid food is begun, introduce one food at a time. This is recommended by La Leche League to help keep the occurrence of allergy at a minimum. By allowing several days between the introduction of each new food, you can watch for any unusual symptoms, such as diarrhea or rash, which may be an indication that the baby is not ready to start that particular food yet.

It is difficult to speak with authority (no matter who you are) about what foods are best. However, some common elements do emerge. Eat foods that are tampered with as little as possible, that is, organically grown, preservative-free, and unrefined. Refined flour, sugar, and salt deplete the body of its resources of vitamins and minerals. Despite the labels claiming that such foods are enriched, they do not contain nearly the nutriments that are present in the whole food products. The presence of bran, for example, in whole wheat becomes essential as roughage. Remember what you made paste with when you were young? White flour and water. Paste literally gums up the works: the longer these refined products stay in the body, the greater the chance that they will putrify in the intestines, creating food for bacteria. It is not yet known what possible functional problems could develop over a lifetime of consuming unnatural foods. Readings from both the area of anthropology and nutrition have led me to think there may be a connection between the consumption of refined food and what Dr. Mike Samuels, in *The Well Body Book*, calls "end-stage disease." By this term he means illnesses that do not produce noticeable symptoms until they have a foothold, but are most likely to have developed over a lifetime of poor habits. The subject of the relationship of health and food additives cannot be discussed in depth here. However, it should be emphasized that no chemical or drug can truly be proven safe.

In relation to the topic of dread disease, a look at one of the worst polio epidemics in North Carolina (1948) is illuminating. Dr. Benjamin Sandler made public announcements concerning the need to control the epidemic by changes in diet. He suggested fresh fruits and vegetables to replace all sugar products. Because all other medical efforts had failed in retarding the epidemic, the public was willing to try anything. Within three days, a significant decline occurred, and the epidemic was under control within a few weeks. The following year polio was down 90 percent in North Carolina.

Exercise. In addition to helping one feel accomplished, physical exercise provides muscle tone. Some health experts say that when sweat glands open, another channel is provided for the elimination of waste matter.

Relaxation. Relaxation and rest have been the hardest for me to realize and therefore something to which I have given a lot of thought. The body needs rest, not only to refuel for future activity but also to allow the body to detoxify. The liver in particular works best to purify the bloodstream when the body is in a state of rest. The "bad breath" after a night's sleep is a sign that it is doing its job. I can often tell when my children are feeling less than par by the change in the smell of their breath.

By taking a half-hour rest period, you are doing a lot to restore your physical and emotional well-being. Techniques such as progressive relaxation, meditation, or Tai Chi, which stress total relaxation, are helpful in promoting good health. Epidemics seem to flourish during periods of great stress. That is, when conditions are poor, whether due to an inadequate physical, social, or psychological environment, disease is more able to take hold. All of us have stress in our lives; the important thing is to develop ways of dealing with it.

Positive Attitude. Not too long ago a friend and I were talking about the difficulty of trying to figure out all the do's and don'ts of healthful living. She commented that her aunt had just died of cancer at the age of 40. The aunt had been meticulous about food and did not indulge in habits such as smoking or drinking, and yet she was, my friend testifies, the grouchiest person she ever knew. An important part of body ecology is joy in living. I feel that the one or two colds a year that I have are often the result of a need to "purge" myself of negative feelings. Without a positive emotional center, it may be hard to realize long-term good health. Going through the process of discovering your own particular diet, exercise, and rest needs, you inevitably develop a new respect for yourself, or as is popular to say, you become more in tune with yourself. Respecting yourself is the first step towards respecting others. Isn't that the seed for a positive way of living? I try to laugh a little every day. Norman Cousins has documented the therapeutic effect of laughter for dread diseases, most notably in his books *Anatomy of an Illness* and *The Healing Heart.* Laughter is jogging for the soul.

Alternative Health Care. I take a vigilant attitude when we are ill. A quiet, restful environment along with time and a lot of tender loving care allows recovery from many illnesses. I have also found that increasing my knowledge of ancient healing disciplines and consulting with professionals trained in alternative healing have been extremely beneficial at times. For example, there are homeopathic remedies that bolster immunity and those that are designed to hasten the cure of specific illnesses. Both professional massage and the kind we share with friends and family members can produce dramatic results. My daughter once gave me such a penetrating massage on the appropriate pressure point that the excrutiating pain I was having from a dry socket (as a result of a wisdom tooth extraction) disappeared, and I was able to get my first night's sleep after days of discomfort. There are other healing disciplines that deserve consideration, and information about them is becoming more accessible.

We are not islands but live in a world where most people are immunized. This changes our native environment. For example, measles used to be endemic; it was a virus that was ever-present. The exposure now is greatly reduced; most children are immunized against it. Because the medical community claims only 85 percent effectiveness, the virus has not been eradicated but simply occurs more rarely in the environment. Being an "unfamiliar" virus, I believe it causes more acute cases of measles than it did when it was a more familiar virus. Consider that in

Africa polio is endemic. The children get it quite commonly (as we do influenza) and without any dire consequences such as paralysis.

The decision to immunize or not is yours. Often when I express my doubts to others about the inoculation procedure, they think I am advocating illness. Instead, what I am advocating is that we find more effective ways of dealing with the sicknesses that plague our culture. It is sad when the older segment in a society becomes subject to so many chronic diseases—arthritis, obesity, diabetes, heart disease, or cancer. But it is even more distressing when these diseases affect children to the extent that they do in present-day America. Cancer is the number one killer of *children*. Our unnatural lifestyle is taking its toll.

I am the mother of two, not a doctor, or a bacteriologist, or a nutritionist. However, as a parent I have a responsibility to get my children off to as good a start in life as possible. Although I do not have access to the laboratory or even the highly technical language of the professional, I nevertheless have questions about countless procedures that are being used in the healthcare arena. I have raised more questions than I have answered. Fortunately, a lot of professionals have started to ask many of these same questions. Still, the thought that continues to trouble me is: What about the questions we haven't thought to ask?

Sources

Bieler, Henry G., MD, and Maxine Block. *Food Is Your Best Medicine.* New York: Ballantine, 1987.

Davis, Adelle. *Let's Have Healthy Children.* New York: NAL, 1981.

Jacobs, Leonard. "Eating Well—The Best Vaccine," "Childhood Illnesses," "Natural Pediatrics." *Mothering*, no. 9 (Fall 1978): 17–24.

Kloss, Jethro. *Back to Eden.* Loma Linda, CA: Promise Books, 1989.

McBean, Eleanor. *The Poisoned Needle.* Mokelumne Hill, CA: Health

Research, 1974.

Mendelsohn, Robert, MD. (Interview). *East West Journal* (October 1978). *The People's Doctor* Newsletter.

Samuels, Mike, MD, and Hal Z. Bennett. *The Well Body Book.* New York: Random house,1973.

Shelton, Herbert M., MD. *The Hygienic System.* Mokelumne Hill, CA: Health Research, 1956.

Well Being, no. 7.

CODY'S REACTION

Dear *Mothering*,

Since the birth of our son, Cody (now 19 months), we have tried to make the correct decision about whether or not to immunize. Around two weeks before each shot date, my husband, John, and I discuss it—going back and forth on the decision—and then finally decide, yes, it's the right thing for his protection.

Well, when Cody had his MMR shot (at 16 months), his reaction brought an extreme awareness to us. When I signed the consent paper saying I knew that one in a million has a post-vaccinal encephalitis reaction, I did not possibly believe that

my son would be that *one!*

My little one could not handle the poison from the shot. Ten days after the shot, he was feverish, went into convulsions, was in a stupor, and did not breathe for three minutes! I cannot describe the fear, the panic-state that I was in. My friend Melinda raced us, running stop lights, to the emergency room. I gave Cody mouth-to-mouth resuscitation on the way, which I could barely think how to do. My child was dying. A couple of times his eyes rolled back into his head and then came back out searching my eyes for help. I was so freaked out that I shook his blue, weightless body, pleading, "Please Cody, breathe, breathe . . . come back."

I ran into the emergency room yelling, "This child is not breathing!" Just then Cody gasped and started crying. He turned pink and then pale. He had a temperature of 104° and very swollen glands (the mumps reaction). His fever lasted for 30 hours after that. John and I were by his side, sponging him, holding him, listening for his breath, crying, praying, thankful that he was alive, and wishing the whole thing were over and we had a healthy child again. Three days later he broke out with a measles rash.

It has been a couple of months now since the reaction. I shall never forget it! Not one moment of it.

I have done extensive research lately on the whole immunization business. *Mothering* has been very helpful in providing addresses for informa-tion. Eleanor McBean is one author who has very thorough information on the subject.

I now have the whole picture—both sides! I have made my decision not to poison my child again (John agrees). I have a lot of proof to back up my decision, and I'm ready to face any type of feedback . . . and boy does it take courage! I realize that the decision to immunize is totally up to the parents, and I'm not going to be pushy on anyone. I only urge people to find out about both sides before making a decision!

I love your magazine from front to back—every issue. You are inspiring, and you are doing excellent work!

Yours for health and
happiness,
Dana Reaves

IF IMMUNIZATIONS DO WORK . . .

Dear American Medical Association,

Simple logic has brought me to a few too many questions concerning vaccinations. There are no answers to be found through the health division; Lester F. Cour, Oregon Immunization Program, to whom I've written previously, has avoided answering my questions specifically.

1) If immunizations do work, if they aren't harmful and they are safe, then why are they repeated? Why aren't they guaranteed, and why were 100,000 DPT serums being located and disposed of?

From Washington, DC (Associated Press): "The government announced the recall Wednesday of more than 100,000 doses of vaccine designed to protect from diphtheria, whooping cough, and tetanus following the deaths of four babies within 24 hours after receiving the vaccine. . . ."

The deaths originally appeared to have resulted from the little-understood Sudden Infant Death Syndrome (SIDS), also known as crib death.

The government said the Tennessee Health Department noticed a possible connection between one lot of Wyeth vaccine and the sudden deaths of eight infants. But it took no immediate action until it realized early this month that four of the deaths had occurred within 24 hours of a DPT vaccination.

No immediate action was taken "because DPT vaccine is generally administered for the first time at two months of age—precisely the age when the risk of sudden, unexplained death is greatest for infants. . . ."

2) Why are adverse reactions kept hush-hush?

3) Why in underdeveloped countries, where immunization programs are used (for example, India), do we still see disease so widespread? This would lead me to think that hygiene, sanitation, and diet are of utmost importance in preventing disease.

4) If 600 people are unimmunized and 6 get polio, is this because they were *not* immunized? If 600 people are immunized and 6 get polio, is this because they *were* immunized?

I am not sold on the idea that injecting a disease into my healthy son would improve his health.

There is so little anti-immunization literature available. Where is the truth? Somehow, after the swine flu fiasco, I had the feeling I wasn't told the whole truth!

Thank you,
Layah Rutledge

A MOTHER RESEARCHES IMMUNIZATION

Roxanne Bank

"A Mother Researches Immunization" first appeared in Mothering, *no. 16 (Summer 1980).*

This is a pro *and* con article on immunization. I wish to offer some information in addition to that which *Mothering* has already published and to correct potentially dangerous misinformation included in the articles in *Mothering* (Fall 1978) by Leonard Jacobs ("Eating Well—The Best Vaccine," "Childhood Illnesses," and "Natural Pediatrics")[1] so that concerned parents can make rational choices about vaccination.

I believe that illness indicates an imbalance within a person's inner environment that can be affected by conditions in the external world. It is possible to maintain a balance—to eat properly, exercise regularly, and think positively—and to have a pure body, mind, and spirit even in this polluted, imbalanced environment. We have this power, but we rarely use it. It is *not* possible to maintain such a balance in someone else, for example one's child, without full cooperation of the other person. I will not debate the germ theory. Suffice it to say that people do get sick when they are susceptible—*somehow!*

One may have complete faith in divine perfection and be willing to accept health or illness within one's family as God's will and to take responsibility for such a stand and its ramifications. I have no argument with such a position.

I believe that, as Jacobs says, "modern society, with its artificial environment and diet may be a significant factor in the cause of modern sicknesses." Human beings are far removed from living in harmony with the natural order. Immunizations are antithetical to the natural order, which allows for survival of the fittest, because they work against the natural elimination of weaker humans through disease. If you favor following the natural order, you might not choose immunization but might, therefore, some day watch your child experience crippling illness or death. If you do choose immunization, you may watch your child experience illness or death anyway—maybe sooner.

Even if we improve our diets and change our home environments, we still live in the modern polluted world where people smoke cigarettes and produce chemical waste matter.

Serious questions concerning the long-term effects of standardly accepted injectable toxins on the body (whether they collect in certain areas in the body or whether they increase the system's susceptibility to other diseases like cancer or heart disease) can only be clearly evaluated over a period of many years of observing immunized persons and related studies. To the best of my knowledge, thorough studies of this nature are not yet available. However, I can say that I personally know of one case in which serious illness was traced to the accumulation of vaccinated toxins in certain areas of the person's body. This is a consideration.

There are many unknowns still. Without debating all the issues, I offer some helpful information.

I believe two important factors are involved in disease—the balance or imbalance of the body and the exposure to dangerous bacteria or viruses. In his letter (*Mothering*, Summer 1979) Victor LaCerva makes the important point that "if a period of susceptibility is matched with exposure to a given virus or bacteria, disease may result."[2] Leonard Jacobs neglects this point and fails to discuss the fact that although most human bodies survive most infectious diseases ("discharge" them), varying amounts of damage—reversible or irreversible—can occur (brain damage, paralysis). And while he denounces the germ theory, Jacobs suggests that we expose our maturing offspring "to a wide variety of stimuli and possible 'germs' in order to elicit the production of antibodies which will give lasting immunity to sickness." What he is, in fact, recommending is that we expose our children to *live* virulent viruses rather than exposing them to dead or subdued viruses via immunizations! He insinuates that the risk is *less* because it's "natural" and that our bodies will somehow stay purer this way. Please remember there are many "natural" poisons in our environment, and use of herbs should be undertaken with sincere respect for their potency. Herbs can kill. And please be aware that *chemical* is not necessarily a bad word. You and I and your favorite herbal tea are made up of chemicals!

Jacobs points out that he presents only his own opinions; he provides no factual data to support his statements and even says that no studies exist from which to evaluate the effectiveness of immunization. This is simply not true.

Some corrections of other errors included in Jacobs's articles are these:

1) Tetanus is *not* an "infectious" disease in the sense that it is contagious, although it is an infection to the body.

2) Polio, tetanus, and diphtheria are prevalent among children but are *not only childhood diseases*. Therefore, it is important for us to realize that adults are directed to get booster vaccinations every 10 years for these diseases.[3]

3) Some vaccinations *have* been proven to provide immunity. For example, tetanus: "During the Civil War, 205 cases of tetanus occurred for every 100,000 wounds. This rate was reduced to 16 per 100,000 wounds in World War I, presumably as a result

of better surgical care of wounds and liberal use of tetanus anti-toxin prepared in horses. By World War II, all United States military personnel were required to accept tetanus toxoid; among more than 2.5 million injuries only 12 cases of tetanus occurred, of whom 8 had not been adequately immunized. This rate of 0.44 cases of tetanus per 100,000 wounded represents a 99.8 percent reduction from the Civil War."[4] Jacobs comments on the rarity of tetanus in this country, intimating that vaccination is therefore unnecessary. However, the primary reason for the rarity is vaccination! In the civilian population, 102 cases of tetanus were recorded in the United States in 1975; 45 of them were fatal;[5] " . . . in all of these individuals tetanus immunization had never been given, was incomplete or was unknown."[6]

4) Jacobs implies that improvement in sanitary conditions and food handling are the *primary* reasons for the reduction in infectious diseases. "To a considerable extent in some diseases, the decline in mortality can be attributed to people's intervention in terms of sanitary control of water supply and refuse and proper food handling. An example . . . is typhoid fever."[7] Deaths due to salmonella (food poisoning) have also declined for these reasons. Other factors influencing improvement in health of the general population include quarantine measures (diminished incidence of tuberculosis); control of nonhuman vectors (animals), which has affected the decline of rabies, typhus fever, and malaria; improved nutrition; and changes in socioeconomic and educational status. Therefore, in the case of a number of diseases (cholera, plague, typhoid fever) "immunization . . . has been of negligible importance [and] is reserved for those who, because of occupation or travel, cannot avoid exposure."[8]

However, "the disappearance of mortality from one disease (smallpox) and the rarity of deaths from two others (tetanus and polio) can be attributed almost entirely to active immunization . . . with no other factors seeming to exert influence. . . . The decline in measles mortality is a result of at least two factors. . . . For reasons unknown, mortality rates declined from approximately 10 per 100,000 population during the years 1912 to 1918 to less than 0.3 per 100,000 in the 1950s before licensure of the vaccine. Since licensure, annual attack rates from measles have decreased precipitously to less than 20 per 100,000, and deaths to less than 0.01 per 100,000."[9] The value of immunization should not be measured only in terms of lives saved: "For Massachusetts during the years 1965–1971, it was estimated that measles immunization efforts prevented more than 114,000 of 137,000 cases that would have been expected without immunization, thus averting 10 deaths and 114 cases of encephalitis, of whom ⅓ would have been expected to incur permanent intellectual impairment. The ultimate saving in healthcare costs in Massachusetts was estimated at $5.5 million."[10]

5) This information contradicts the insinuation by Jacobs that "self-interest and economic ties" influence decisions made by doctors and research scientists. Personally, I agree that doctors and pharmacists who are primarily interested in financial gain do exist. Medicine *is* big business, and usually it is run competitively and expensively rather than cooperatively and efficiently. However, there are also American Medical Association (AMA) doctors who are evolving toward holistic healing, back to family practice, and who emphasize to their patients and to the public through advertising the importance of good nutrition and exercise in

preventing disease. To be fair, we need to remember that even though doctors advocate preventive medicine, their patients often do not *practice* preventive measures.

In conclusion, I would like to comment on several general points concerning vaccination. First, evidence has shown that giving several vaccines at the same time is safe, although "combining individual vaccines from different manufacturers into one shot cannot be recommended."[11] One may choose not to get all of what is available or to get chosen inoculations one at a time in order to minimize side effects or to be able to verify the source of specific side effects. "Prolonged time between the injections of basic series of diphtheria-tetanus does not interfere with the final immunity."[12]

Second, since breastfeeding provides some measure of immunity, one may choose to delay immunization beyond the age recommended by the Department of Health, Education and Welfare. If vaccinations are your choice, it would be wise to make sure that your child is not ill or teething in order to minimize side effects. Taking vitamins (especially vitamin C) for several days prior to getting shots probably would be helpful.

At this point our 21-month-old son has had no immunizations. He will never get shots for mumps, rubella, or pertussis. We are still debating the other inoculations. Although we favor following the natural order as much as we can, that is sometimes not possible. If we had followed the natural process during childbirth, my son and I would have died. (His head was transverse and at 9 pounds, 1 ounce I could not push him out. He was delivered with forceps in a hospital after 16 hours of hard labor at home.) It has been several generations since most of our families followed the natural order. After evolving away from this natural order, we should be careful how we return to it. My guess is that many of us are not as hardy as our ancestors. It seems to me that the proper path would be to combine the best of what technology offers with the best aspects of simple living in harmony with our environment. We do not have all the answers, but we are learning together as we go. In my heart I believe that each of us—whatever our frame of reference—is doing what we believe is best and most loving. We all have our blind spots. We all need love and patience.

Notes

1. Leonard Jacobs, "Eating Well—The Best Vaccine," "Childhood Illnesses," "Natural Pediatrics," *Mothering*, no. 9 (Fall 1978): 17–24.
2. Victor LaCerva (letter), *Mothering*, no. 12 (Summer 1979): 87–88.
3. United States Department of Health Immunization Schedule, vol. 12, p. 87.
4. Edward A. Mortimer, Jr., "Immunization against Infectious Disease," *Science 200* (26 May 1978): 905.
5. *Parents' Guide to Childhood Immunization*, United States Department of Health, Education and Welfare, Public Health Service (October 1977), p. 17.
6. See Note 4, p. 905.
7. Ibid., p. 904.
8. Ibid.
9. Ibid.
10. Ibid.
11. Carol F. Phillips, MD, "Children Out of Step with Immunization," *Pediatrics for the Clinician* (11 November 1974): 880.
12. Ibid.

MORE ON IMMUNIZATIONS

Dear Editors:

As a pediatrician, I have appreciated *Mothering*'s raising of people's consciousness about many of the things we physicians do "on automatic" in medicine. Minds *can* be opened and stretched.

Because of my training in Western medicine, I am obviously a biased mother, and yet I also agonized over the decision to vaccinate our children. The smallpox vaccination, which was still required when our kids were young, was hardest for me. Finally, the public schools "caught" me and with much fear and trepidation, my children's immunizations were completed in order for them to enter first grade. But I felt somehow deprived of my rights in decision making for my children.

Since then, my family and I have had a unique experience that I would like to share. We moved to a developing area of the world, where my husband and I practiced medicine, and where 80 beautiful breastfed babies would come in yearly to die of tetanus. This was an area where babies who had never had a single canned, frozen, or processed morsel of food would die by droves of whooping cough, and where little children who had never had an antibiotic would suffocate with their diphtheritic membranes. It seemed to us that only the cute little kids got polio. Measles, though, was different; rubella usually killed the sickly.

I am not writing this to frighten readers, but only to say that I would have been much more casual today about immunizations had it not been for the day-to-day reality of living in an area where these diseases are present. You could cite the outbreak of polio among the Amish here, I suppose—they are well known for pure living and contracted polio last August. Or the history of diphtheria epidemics in southern New Mexico—Marie Hughes remembered one village that lost *all* boys under two years of age one year while she was a leader and parents were still frightened of vaccines.

My kids, had they been unimmunized and living in the United States, probably wouldn't have gotten these communicable diseases, but not because I am such a good cook of natural foods and rarely use antibiotics. The reason would have been simply that the disease reservoir is low here. That is not to say that breastfeeding, sound nutrition, and the cautious use of medicines aren't all important, too. But we can't lose sight of the real factor: exposure.

We need to give thanks to the generation who went ahead of us and immunized their children so ours may live at a time of little exposure. Do we have a responsibility to future generations to keep the pool of disease down? I think so. As with smallpox, once the pool for any disease gets small enough, then the vaccination will be unnecessary and we will all be winners.

Most parents are concerned about the possibility of dangerous reactions to immunizations, and their concern is legitimate, of course. More development of even safer immunizations can and should be done. We could be a force for insisting that manufacturers of the vaccine for pertussis, for example, continue to refine and improve their product. Why not write to:

Wyeth Laboratories
Professional Services
PO Box 8299
Philadelphia, PA 19101

Lederle Laboratories
Customer Service
7611 Carpenter Freeway
Dallas, TX 75247

Connaught Laboratories
Customer Service
PO Box 187
Swiftwater, PA 18370
and tell them you are not satisfied. Ask if they are devoting research time and money to the improvement of their vaccines. Perhaps, too, a letter to your health departments (local and state) would be effective, as they are the largest purchasers of vaccines. You might also ask why the United States pertussis vaccine is different from the World Health Organization recommendations (*New England Journal of Medicine 303*, no. 3, 1980, p. 157).

I think the question of the safety of immunizations is a very important one. But I have lived with and witnessed the danger of not immunizing in today's world.

I suppose, too, I am more deeply concerned about what I see as an even greater threat to children's health these days— a threat against which we cannot immunize. And that is nuclear war. Maybe it is time that we concerned parents move on to tackle what may really ruin our children's lives: an uninhabitable planet.

Sue Brown, MD
Albuquerque, NM

ON IMMUNIZATION

Daniel A. Lander, DC

Dr. Daniel A. Lander has a family chiropractic practice in Coopers Mills, Maine. He has written and lectured on vaccination, nutrition, and chiropractic work. An earlier version of "On Immunization" appeared in Mothering, no. 21 (Fall 1981).

The practice of immunization in the United States has, for the most part, been accepted without opposition. The public has been intimidated by scare tactics and guilt either to immunize their children or be labeled negligent parents.

The truth is that immunization practices in this country are not as cut-and-dried as assumed. The practice of medicine today is designed to intervene with nature, replacing natural logic and function with scientific logic and practices. The approach is to try and eliminate the offending causes of diseases, such as bacteria or viruses. And as necessary as that may be at times, the promotion of health may be a better preventive alternative.

The fluoride issue is a good example. Fluoride was thought to be an effective treatment in decreasing the number of dental cavities in children. This knowledge was implemented by fluoridating our drinking water. On the surface, this seems like a good idea, until we think about the real causes of tooth decay. The causes vary—from improper nutrition or oral hygiene to genetics or other factors. However, lack of fluoride is not a cause. Fluoridating drinking water is a means of treating the symptom rather than the cause of the problem.

Another solution to the problem of tooth decay and probably many other diseases may be the promotion and maintenance of health. This solution may be more rewarding and more effective, for the human body is a complex piece of organic machinery that knows how to restore and maintain health. The human body makes adrenalin, antibiotics, insulin, pain relievers, vitamins, and even drugs that have not been discovered yet. There is a wisdom within the body that builds and maintains it, and this wisdom created each of us from one solitary cell within a mother's womb. Miraculously, from one cell, the combination of the sperm and egg, the 35 quadrillion cells of the body are formed and then organized into a living machine, with all the parts capable of performing specific functions for total body unity. The human body is usually taken for granted, and not fully appreciated unless one stops and thinks about it. The wisdom that created our bodies is far superior to the finite minds of all scientists in the world.

This short article is not intended to influence decisions about whether or not parents should vaccinate their children, but to inform people of the risks and hazards involved in artificial immunization. The following excerpts are from articles published within the last 16 years and represent some research and opinions that oppose mass immunization. These statements point out that there is not as yet a definitive answer to the immunization question, and no one knows for sure how effective or safe immunization really is:

Cholera, dysentery and typhoid (similarly) peaked and dwindled outside the physician's control. The combined death rate from scarlet fever, diphtheria, whooping cough and measles among children up to fifteen shows that nearly 90% of the total decline in mortality between 1860 and 1965 had occurred before the introduction of antibiotics and widespread immunization. —Ivan Illich, Medical Nemesis *(New York: Random House, 1976).*

At a recent conference at Tufts University, Alec Burton, O.D., said no one will deny the existence of germs and other micro-organisms, or that they are intimately associated with certain diseases. They may be secondary or tertiary factors, but they are not the primary and funda-mental causes of diseases. They are intimately associated with, and nec-essary to, the evolution of some diseases, but condition of the host is the primary factor.

The human body has the ability to resist almost all types of organisms or toxins that tend to damage the tissues and organs. This capacity is called immunity. —*Arthur C. Guyton,* Textbook of Medical Phys-iology *(Philadelphia: W. B. Saunders Co., 1976), p. 77.*

One of the best arguments against immunization is the swine flu vaccination program. A look at this program might give us some insight into whether or not we have learned anything about immunization practices:

The singular death of an already sick Army private necessitates a flu vaccine program for the entire country, despite the evidence that it is not solely the virus that really makes one ill; it is the combination of the virus and a body incapable of adapting to that particular organism. By injecting that very organism into an individual who isn't 100% healthy, are you going to increase the capabilities of his body, or is there a greater chance that you directly cause even more physiological harm by this added stress? When you're dealing with a system as totally com-plex as our biological one, you better let people decide for themselves just what they want to put into their bodies. As a newspaper writer so aptly put it—it was as if Mother Nature were warning us against arrogance; there are many things in a world full of biological hazards that we don't understand, don't even have the tools to understand. —Richard Knox, "A Shot in the Arm, a Shot in the Dark," Boston Sunday Globe *(26 December 1976).*

Not only may vaccinations produce such adverse effects as producing the very disease that they are intended to prevent, not only may they cause a variety of unhealthy side effects, or even other diseases, but when they work properly, their results are far inferior to the perfect work of a healthy body. In fact, if one is weak to begin with, they hesitate to inoculate at all since that added stress may be the very catalyst to make one sick or even dead. —A. M. Prince, *"Our Last Vaccine?"* Science *(28 March 1977): 9.*

One of the most controversial points of the immunization controversy is the polio vaccine. What about it? Many people object to some of the vaccines, but feel the polio vaccine is an absolute must. What if these same people knew the following:

L. A. Times Service—*On May 8, 1970, at the Hidalgo County Public Health Mission, Texas, a registered nurse administered two drops of Sabin oral polio vaccine to Anita Reyes, then eight months old. Two weeks later, Anita was hospitalized with an illness that resembled a bad case of influenza with the added complication of weakness in her legs. Tests soon confirmed the later suspicion that she had polio. . . .*

Anita's immunization had been routine, and the polio vaccine was determined not to be defective. In fact, Anita was one of a small but significant number of apparently healthy Americans who contract paralytic poliomyelitis each year from apparently normal vaccine . . . figures released by the federal Centers for Disease Control (CDC) in Atlanta show that the oral vaccine used almost universally in the world today has, in the United States, become the dominant cause of polio. —Philadelphia Inquirer *(25 November 1976).*

Four medical scientists told a Senate hearing yesterday that the oral polio vaccine has caused nearly all of the few reported cases of poliomyelitis since 1961 and is riskier than no vaccine at all.

Dr. Jonas Salk, discoverer of the killed virus vaccine, testified that the live-virus vaccine, discovered by Dr. Albert Sabin, was "the principal if not the sole cause of the 140 polio cases reported in the U. S. since 1961.

"At the present time the risk of acquiring polio from the live-virus vaccine is greater than from naturally occurring viruses," he told the Senate Health Subcommittee.

All of the scientists criticized the form on which the parents now give public health officials "informed consent" to treat their children with live vaccine. They acknowledge neither the risk nor the existence of the alternate killed virus, they said. —Washington Post *(24 September 1976).*

I would like to point out that the information reported in these articles might only be the tip of the iceberg compared to what may be discovered in the future. Let us see what we know about the long-term effects of immunization.

Viruses May Leave Hidden Specter

Rutgers University microbiologists in St. Petersburg Beach, Florida, are investigating the possibility that viruses acquired during childhood through vaccination may silently survive in the body long after the original infection is gone, according to a Washington Star *news report.*

The vaccinations under suspicion are the live-virus type, not the dead virus that will be used in the pending massive swine flu inoculation.

Normally, this reservoir of genetic material found in the live virus might help maintain long immunity to further infections. But the "hidden specter" in harboring such viruses is that they also may play a role in triggering the onset of human cancer or rare chronic degenerative diseases such as multiple sclerosis.

This research raises questions about the possible risks associated with widespread use of live-virus vaccines in the prevention of measles, mumps, polio and other infectious diseases. —I.C.A. Review *(July 1976).*

Upper respiratory infections are perhaps the most common risk of vaccination. There is no doubt in my mind that immunizing children at two to six months of age is the largest cause of upper respiratory infections, allergies, and ear infections. A little common sense would indicate what mothers know: that infants should not get egg albumin or other such proteins before four to six months of age. Yet mothers will allow children to be injected with a potent foreign protein because it is called "immunization." —Dr. Daniel A. Lander, Immunization: An Informed Choice *(1978).*

In summary, here are some of the problems of artificial immunization:

■ Statistics regarding the effectiveness of various vaccines are very subjective.

■ They can cause the disease itself, or other health problems.

■ Your body's own "acquired immunity" lasts a lifetime, requiring no "booster shots."

■ Political-medical-corporate overtones characterize every vaccination program.

■ The experts themselves disagree on specific modes of dispersal.

■ The overwhelming majority of people successfully adapt to viruses when they come into contact with them naturally in the environment.

One may wonder if there is not a more natural and less dangerous alternative. Indeed, there is: strengthen the adaptive capabilities of your own body. When it is working right it may be the first line of defense for health. Eating good food, exercising regularly, living in a clean environment, and experiencing relative peace of mind all enable your body to maintain its homeostasis with the environment.

You have a choice regarding immunization. If you decide not to immunize your child but are concerned with legal ramifications within the school, let your state and federal legislators know your position—that you would at least like a choice!

IMMUNIZATIONS AND INFORMED CONSENT

Carol Miller

Carol Miller is a public health consultant and rural health advocate. She is currently focusing her legislative advocacy work on the development of healthcare policies and congressional support to assure that the needs of the underserved are considered in the development of any type of national healthcare reform. An earlier version of "Immunizations and Informed Consent" appeared in Mothering, *no. 26 (Winter 1983).*

This article is not a scientific analysis of the information available about immunizations. It describes the research I have done and also teaches how to do computer searches for information, but primarily shares the conclusions I have drawn about current United States immunization policy after five years of studying the question.

I first began to research the issue of immunization in 1976 because of the swine flu vaccine. I was in Berkeley at the School of Public Health studying for a master's degree, and all of our classes emphasized the importance of the swine flu vaccine. When it became apparent that the vaccine was not only a total failure, but was also a health hazard and killer, there was a great deal of embarrassment among the vaccine proponents on the faculty.

My interest in immunizations has continued since then, and I have researched the issue in numerous medical journals. I feel compelled to write this article to help parents sift through the vast number of conflicting reports in order to decide whether or not they should immunize their children.

Laws about Health

The worst thing about the United States immunization policy is that it is law. In 49 states it is mandatory for children to be immunized in order to attend school. Wyoming is the only state without such a law, but that is because it has the highest *voluntary* immunization rate in the country. There are schedules of specific immunizations by certain ages that *must* be met by all children . . . or must they?

It is possible for parents to file as conscientious objectors with their state health department, although this choice is not

advertised. Several people I know who are conscientious objectors state that it is their "God-given right to refuse to immunize
their child." Any lesser statement is unacceptable legally. For
example, it is unacceptable legally to say, "I read 25 articles in
medical journals, three newspaper articles, and saw on the
"Today" show that the pertussis vaccine has serious side effects,
and for this reason I don't want my child to have the pertussis
vaccine." Such a statement is not reason enough from a legal
standpoint to refuse to immunize your child against pertussis.
This is one of the most serious problems with immunization policy; in order to legally refuse any single immunization it is necessary to be opposed to all immunizations on religious grounds.
Scientific evidence against the effectiveness of particular immunizations is insufficient. A court case may be necessary to test
this discrepancy.

The Scientific Evidence

The particular computer search I did turned up 161 articles
about health problems associated with immunizations, and all
of these articles were only for the years 1980 and 1981. There
is a tremendous debate in the medical world about the dangers
of immunizations, but none of this information is leaked to the
public until a large number of tragedies occur. The scientific
evidence exists against some immunizations, but the political
and economic reasons for their continuation remain stronger
than these facts.

Informed Consent

Informed consent is an elusive concept, one which is often

only resolved in courts of law. In the area of immunizations, there is almost no such thing as informed consent. Parents must sign a release of liability to the drug company when giving their child the polio vaccine because so many victims have suffered from the treatment that the company is forced to protect itself. There is very little accurate information being presented about the other vaccines.

What is known about vaccines is an entirely different story from what is told. Healthcare consumers should insist on reading the package inserts that come with vaccines. Many medical professionals have never read these inserts and therefore are not able to tell you that there are some conditions that make vaccines health hazards.

Although the actual package inserts detail the very serious complications of immunizations, the federal Centers for Disease Control (CDC, the agency in charge of national immunization policy) sent a letter to all of the state immunization officers that said:

Vaccine Side Effects—Vaccines are among our safest and most reliable medicines. However, vaccines like many medicines can cause side effects. These are usually mild and brief, such as low fever, sore arm, slight rash, or irritability after taking the shot. Very rarely, they are serious. For this reason, vaccines should be given only by physicians or other qualified persons and only to those who need them.

I would like to contrast this official policy statement of the federal government with a letter I received from a mother as a result of an article I wrote for *New Age* magazine, entitled "The Truth

about Immunizations" (September 1980). I received more letters in response to this article than I have in response to anything else I have ever written. I am overwhelmed by the concern of people about this issue:

Dear Carol,

*Outrage seems like an over-simplified word to use in expressing our
feeling when our perfectly healthy (then 15 ½-month-old) son received
a measles-mumps-rubella shot. Not only did the health department
flyer, explaining the vaccine and its reactions, clearly misinform us, but
the nurse who administered the vaccine was just as ignorant. After less
than 24 hours our warm, smiling, energetic kid turned into a zombie,
burning a fever of close to 105°! The drug company says a reaction to
the shot may occur from 10 to 12 days within the initial administering period. Well somebody ought to set those folks straight and tell them
how our child suffered for close to four days from the vaccine and, on
top of that, on the fifth day broke out in a measly rash which lasted one
and a half weeks.*

Mothering published a similar letter from a mother whose
emotion haunts me as she states, "When I signed the consent paper saying I knew that one in a million has a postvaccinal encephalitis reaction, I did not possibly believe that my son would be that
one!" This letter was also about a reaction to the MMR vaccine.

I could quote many other letters like this and also many more
positive ones from parents all over the country who have refused
to immunize their children. These are satisfied parents with healthy
children who feel that proper diet, breastfeeding, and other lifestyle
choices have helped to make their children healthier than

immunizations could.

Mothering has printed many articles and letters in back issues about the immunization question, but the majority of parents in this country have never learned about the possible hazards. It seems that an organization should be started to educate parents about vaccines and to lobby for their legal right to informed consent.

What Is an Immunization Made of?

Most parents who are trying to feed their children properly would not let them eat a food that contained any of the many ingredients of immunizations. Some of the ingredients in vaccines are: phenol (carbolic acid), formaldehyde (a known cancer causing agent that is commonly used to embalm corpses), mercury (a toxic heavy metal), alum (a preservative), aluminum phosphate (a toxic substance used in deodorants), acetone (a solvent used in fingernail polish remover, very volatile, crosses placenta easily), glycerin, sodium chloride, pig or horse blood, cow pox pus, rabbit brain tissues, dog kidney tissue, monkey kidney tissue, chicken or duck egg protein, and other decomposing protein.

The scientific theory behind immunizations is that by receiving a small dose of a virus or bacteria the body will develop enough immunities to the small dose to protect it from coming down with that specific disease on a larger scale. The animal parts ingredients in immunizations are used to grow the viruses which are later injected into children. The other toxic ingredients are added in either the chemical production of the vaccine or as preservatives.

Foreign Travel and Vaccination

Many people wonder about immunizing their children before traveling to a foreign country. This is a confusing issue with many complicating factors. The most complicating of the factors is that when traveling it is much more difficult for parents to maintain control over their children's environment than it is at home. Food and water may be contaminated, and all living conditions may be unhealthier than at home.

In spite of these difficulties many people travel without receiving immunizations. One of the largest groups to do this is Christian Scientists. Thousands of Christian Scientists travel outside the United States every year, and their religion forbids them to immunize.The Amish and Mennonites are examples of other religious sects that do not believe in vaccination.

How to Make Vaccination Decisions

I stated earlier that this article was not going to be a scientific analysis of immunization. Nor is it a guide to which immunizations to give. This is because of my basic premise that parents have to make decisions for themselves about whether or not to immunize their children and against which diseases. However, I can offer ideas for parents about how to research this issue and where to go for more information. Such information will range from totally provaccination to totally opposed. I am presenting a middle path that encourages parents to learn what they can, ask lots of questions, and then decide what to do for their own child.

Demand informed consent, not only in the matter of immunization, but in any health matter that confronts you. This means you should not agree to any health procedure until all of your questions have been answered to your satisfaction. This is not an easy job, and very few health professionals will help you in your search for answers, but it is a crucial process.

After a while you will be wondering how to know who to believe. Trust your instincts. Don't let guilt prod you into a decision you are uncomfortable with. Locate people whose advice you respect, whether it is newspaper column physician Robert Mendelsohn or "Dear Abby." Magazines like *Mothering, New Age, East West Journal,* and *Yoga Journal* all try to present minority opinions about health issues.

How to Use a Computer to Search for Information

People are drowning in statistics. It seems these days that *any* issue elicits pro and con statistics, and many of us find that too much information can often confuse decision making rather than facilitate it.

Computers have contributed to this because of their incredible information and retrieval capabilities. More people need to learn how to get information from a computer in order to sort out the amount of information with which we are barraged. When I am confused with conflicting information about a health issue, I do a computer search to help make a decision. It is very easy and not too expensive.

There are two ways to do a computer search. With the right tools a search can easily be done on a home or office computer, or the search can be done at a facility with computer search capabilities.

Do-It-Yourself Computer Research

Due to improvements in computer technology and the large number of people who now use computers on a regular basis, obtaining health information is easier than ever. Anyone with a home computer, a modem, and the right software can directly access a variety of electronic data bases and do their own search. People who have a continuing interest in healthcare issues may want to learn how to do their own searches.

The best software to use for medical data searching is GRATE-FUL MED, developed and distributed by the National Library of Medicine at the National Institutes of Health. This software is very easy to use, quite inexpensive, and is available in Macintosh and PC versions. Information about GRATEFUL MED can be obtained from the National Library of Medicine, public information: 800-272-4787, and from MEDLARS Services: 800-638-8480.

Computer Research at a Facility

The second option in computer research is to have it done at a facility. The steps involved in doing such a search follow.

Locate a Facility

Computers that link into health information are located in medical school libraries, hospital libraries, large city libraries, other schools, and at various governmental agencies.

The On-Line Search

Even though it is possible to set up a search over the telephone and receive the results in the mail, if at all possible it is best to be present for the on-line search. On-line means that you are directly linked to the computer and can ask questions, change topics, and see answers immediately as they print out. For example, I did an on-line MEDLINE search on immunization using as key words *failure, poisoning,* and *toxicity.* The computer printed out that there were 1,061 citations. This was too many for the scope of this article so I narrowed it to just *poisoning* and *toxicity* and found that there were 161 citations.

I could have 40 of them printed on-line, so the computer then printed the titles, journals, and issues of the journals on a list for me. This concluded the on-line search. There are a number of other data banks available besides MEDLINE, for example CANLIT for cancer research and TOXLINE for toxicology.

The Off-Line Search

Off-line searches are done on specific retrieval requests and are much cheaper. My on-line search printout with 40 citations cost $9.00, but to have the remaining 121 titles printed out off-line cost only $1.80. Off-line searches are not immediate and may take up to a week.

The Actual Research

Using the same example, the research for this article, I divided the information from the MEDLINE search into categories by type of vaccine. Twenty-two percent of the articles discussed poisoning and toxicity associated with the pertussis immunization, 13 percent with rubella immunization, 9 percent with polio, 7 percent with smallpox, and 6 percent with measles. I decided that 29 of the 121 articles sounded very interesting so before I looked them up in the journals, I did a second off-line search with the identification numbers of those 29 articles in order to have the abstracts (introductions) printed out to study.

This process saves hundreds of research hours. As a health professional I have learned that this journal information is the only data that is considered "worthy" of debate by doctors, so for me it is impossible to skip this step. As a healthcare consumer I have found that the computer search can help me to get better care and change physicians' minds so that others can get better care as well.

PERTUSSIS (WHOOPING COUGH)

Pertussis is an infectious disease of childhood, associated with a specific bacteria. It can sometimes have dramatic and alarming symptoms. Usually it is characterized by a period of cold symptoms followed by an extended period (four to six weeks) of violent coughing. The disease primarily occurs in infants and young children. Deaths from whooping cough are usually due to complicating respiratory infection. Pneumonia is responsible for 90 percent of these deaths in children under three years of age.

In the past ten years 0.4 percent of pertussis cases have proved fatal. The incidence of the disease has steadily decreased in the last 40 years. There were 21,334 cases reported in California in 1941 and only 147 reported in 1980.

Immunity

Little or no immunity is transferred from the mother to the newborn infant. Active immunization with pertussis vaccine is claimed to prevent the disease or lessen the severity of the attack. An attack of the actual disease does not necessarily confer permanent immunity.

Efficacy

The natural history of this disease shows a great reduction in mortality in England long before the vaccine was introduced. Mortality rates continued to decline after the introduction of immunization, but the rate of decline was not significantly greater than before.

Immunization with pertussis vaccine is claimed to induce protective levels of immunity in about 75 percent of those vaccinated. A recent carefully designed but theoretical analysis of pertussis and immunization predicted that the incidence of pertussis would increase 71 times a few years after the cessation of immunizations.

There is conflicting evidence, however, from recent outbreaks of the illness. In one recent report of 8,092 cases of whooping cough, 1,940 (24 percent) were fully immunized and only 2,424 (30 percent) were definitely not immunized. Among 85 fully immunized children studied during an epidemic in 1978, at least 46 developed whooping cough.

Safety

Immunization with pertussis vaccine has been clearly shown to cause a significant number of adverse reactions, some very serious. The most frequent include fevers, behavioral changes (including crying, irritability, and a peculiar screaming syndrome), and redness, swelling, and tenderness at the injection site. A recent carefully conducted study showed that only 7 percent of those receiving the vaccine had no untoward reactions; 54 percent had fevers and 82 percent exhibited behavioral changes.

More serious reactions include encephalitis, convulsions, and brain damage, leading in a sizable number of cases to persistent disease or death. No one is sure how frequently these serious reactions occur; estimates range from 1 in 3,600 to 1 in 500,000. In Britain, during 1969 to 1974 when 64 deaths from whooping cough were reported, there were 56 cases of brain damage following vaccination. In this country, 46 deaths after DPT vaccination were reported in 1979, 33 of them sudden infant deaths. (The pertussis component of the DPT immunization is thought to be responsible for serious reactions following the injection.) It is not clear whether these deaths were caused by the immunization.

In spite of these dangers, the American Academy of Pediatrics has concluded that the benefits of pertussis immunization outweigh the risks. Advocates of immunization say that the risk of convulsions and brain damage following whooping cough is greater than that following vaccination. They also point to a recent significant increase in whooping cough in Great Britain paralleling the decline of immunization as evidence of the necessity for immunization. There is sharp controversy, however, about the reasons for this spread of the disease.

Diagnosis

The characteristic cough of pertussis makes the disease easy to diagnose. The cough comes in paroxysms and is often preceded by a feeling of apprehension or anxiety and tightness in the chest. The cough itself consists of short explosive expirations in rapid succession followed by a long crowing inspiration. During the coughing the child's face may become red or even blue, the eyes bulge, and the tongue protrudes. A number of such paroxysms are sometimes followed by spitting up a mucous plug and vomiting. This will end the attack, and the child will rest or appear dazed. Many of these attacks may occur in one day, more frequently at night and in a stuffy room. They may be brought on by physical exertion, crying, and often by eating and drinking. Attacks diminish when the child is concentrating on toys, books, and so forth. Infants, however, do not always have "whooping" with their cough.

Diagnosis is assisted by identifying the organism (B. pertussis) during the first one or two weeks of illness. After that it becomes difficult to culture the bacteria. High white blood cell counts (20,000 per cu. mm) with a predominance of lymphocytes (60 percent) are characteristic. Complications of pertussis may include cerebral hemorrhage, convulsions, and brain damage, as well as pneumonia, emphysema, or collapsed lung.

Treatment

Standard treatment with antibiotics may help reduce the period of contagion to others and prevent complications. Pertussis immune globula may help shorten the illness and prevent complications and deaths in children under two. Good intensive nursing care is essential.

Summary

Pertussis vaccine is questionably effective and can cause serious side effects in a small number of people. Whooping

cough can be a severe illness, and has in the past resulted in
many deaths, though the percentage of fatalities is now very
low. The ultimate decision and responsibility for immunizing
against pertussis must rest with the child's parents. In general, the clinic does not recommend the administration of this
vaccination.

Excerpted with permission from Immunizations: Are They Necessary?—*a past publication of the Hering Family Health Clinic,
Berkeley, California.*

Carol Miller

CONSTITUTIONAL RIGHTS AND IMMUNIZATION

Officially, immunization policy in the United States comes from two primary sources: the American Academy of Pediatrics and the federal Centers for Disease Control (CDC). These two groups issue guidelines and policies that are used by most healthcare providers and state health departments. However, in reality most immunization policy is either developed by or developed in connection with the vaccine manufacturers. There are varied approaches to the implementation of these policies among states and other public health agencies. Some states and public school districts are much more accepting of parents who object to immunization than others.

Parents in many locales have protested that their rights and their children's rights have been infringed on due to overzealous immunization policies. Children have been threatened with expulsion or ousted from schools for their beliefs—even when these children belonged to a religion that prohibits immunization. There have been cases where social service agencies have taken children away from their parents, called these parents unfit, and forced the children to be immunized. It is sad to report that in many places, authorities treat people who disagree with mainstream immunization policies as if they have no constitutional rights to choose which medical services they want. Those policies are challenged in courts, and various jurisdictions adjudicate them differently.

What interest group has the most rights when it comes to immunizations? It is not surprising that the drug manufacturers have reserved most of these rights for themselves. They develop and manufacture a product that has a gigantic automatic market. And they are completely protected from liability by United States taxpayers.

The case of the pertussis vaccine provides a good illustration of this situation. In the past, numerous children have had adverse reactions to the pertussis vaccine, so many that articles about such cases appeared frequently in newspapers, and parents of affected children were guests on TV talk shows. As a result, many parents began to fear the pertussis vaccine. Then the manufacturer slowed production to a standstill, and suddenly there was a shortage. Rather than reassess the national pertussis immunization policy, the federal government agreed to absolve manufacturers of any liability and established a Vaccine Injury Trust Fund administered by the Department of Health and Human Services (DHHS). This fund provides tax dollars to compensate people injured by vaccines. However, even though the taxpayers now pay for vaccine-caused death and injury, there has been no reduction in the price charged for vaccines. In the 1992 Public Health Service budget (DHHS), the vaccine injury program received $82.5 million. This amount is over and above the millions in the Vaccine Injury Trust Fund. The question remains, if the government has to pay so many millions of dollars every year to compensate people injured by vaccines, why can't parents have the right *not* to immunize their children?

Carol Miller

VACCINATIONS AND IMMUNE MALFUNCTION

Harold E. Buttram and John Chriss Hoffman

Harold E. Buttram, MD, is a general practitioner in addition to specializing in allergy and environmental medicine. He lives in Quakertown, Pennsylvania. John Chriss Hoffman studied for his PhD in microbiology at the Catholic University in Washington, DC, and has been involved in the vaccination debate since 1978. "Vaccinations and Immune Malfunction" first appeared in Mothering, *no. 28 (Summer 1983).*

One of the fundamental issues concerning current vaccination programs can be summarized in the following question: Is there a significant difference between the immunity acquired in the natural course of a disease, such as mumps or measles, and the immunity gained from vaccines? There do appear to be fundamental differences.

Natural immunity in a healthy person is based on a series of body defenses, much like the defenses of a medieval fortified castle. Vaccinations, on the other hand, inject massive amounts of vaccine preparations directly into the body, thus bypassing the outer defenses.

By way of illustration, let us assume that a child is born with a total immune capacity of 100 units. According to the *one cell, one antibody* rule, once an immune body (plasma cell or lymphocyte) becomes committed to a given antigen, it becomes incapable of responding to other antigens or challenges. Again, let us assume that a hypothetical child 20 or more years ago passed through the usual childhood diseases of former decades (measles, mumps, chicken pox, and so on) with relatively minor and uncomplicated illnesses. Considering the extreme efficiency of natural immunity, we may make an educated guess that permanent immunity was gained to these diseases by utilizing only 3 to 7 percent of the total immune capacity. In the case of the routine childhood vaccines, in contrast, it is likely that a higher percentage of the total immune capacity becomes committed, perhaps something on the order of 30 to 70 percent. As noted above, once an immune body becomes committed to a specific antigen, it becomes inert and incapable of responding to other challenges.

If the reserve capacity of children is being reduced by current vaccinations in this manner, what will be the consequences? No one knows for certain at this time, but it is possible that these consequences could be seen as an increased susceptibility to viruses, to other infections, and to various forms of allergies. The effects may be seen as immunologic disorders in the form of *autoimmune diseases*, which are increasingly recognized in modern times. Finally, there is indisputable evidence that many instances of mental and nervous disorders are caused by immunologic aberrations.[1, 2, 3, 4, 5] The relationship of these disorders to vaccinations remains speculative at this time, but there is a substantial and growing body of evidence that modern vaccines can result in immune malfunction.

The Evidence

For many years immunologists have been aware of a state of *anergy* (immunological unresponsiveness) following vaccinations. For example, live-virus vaccines have been shown to transiently suppress tuberculin sensitivity.[6, 7]

One of the most extensively documented studies of the indirect effects of vaccines is to be found in the book *The Hazards of Immunization*[8] by Sir Graham Wilson, formerly of the Public Health Laboratory Service, England and Wales. In his chapter entitled "Indirect Effects: Provocation Disease," Dr. Wilson provides a number of documented historical examples in which vaccination against one disease seemed to provoke another. As one example, a physician in London first drew attention to the relation between inoculations against diphtheria or pertussis and attacks of poliomyelitis when he described 15 cases he had seen between 1944 and 1949. Paralysis came on, as a rule, seven to 21 days after injection and affected the left arm, into which injections were usually given, four times as often as the right. In describing this type of occurrence, Wilson stated:

When a vaccine is injected into the tissues during the incubation period of a disease or during the course of a latent infection, it may bring on an acute attack of the disease. That is to say, the incubation period is shortened, or a latent infection that might have given rise to no manifest illness is converted into a clinical attack. The two diseases in which this so-called provocation effect has been most studied are typhoid fever and poliomyelitis, but evidence exists to show that it may be operative in other diseases.

An important investigation into the role of malnutrition and vaccination as causative factors in immune dysfunction has been in progress among the Australian aborigines since the early 1970s by Archie Kalokerinos, MD, of New South Wales, Australia (later aided by Glen Dettman, PhD, Orthomolecular Medisearch, of Mentone, Australia).

One of the first published reports of large-scale immune malfunction following the conventional childhood vaccines is to be found in the book *Every Second Child*[9] by Archie Kalokerinos. In this book, Dr. Kalokerinos describes his work as a physician in the 1960s and 1970s among Australian aborigines. In early work with these peoples, he was appalled by the high infant mortality rate—death rates in some areas having soared to 50 percent.

The Australian aborigines were a unique population: they lacked the natural resistance to many infectious diseases to which the Caucasian race has been exposed through the centuries. Moreover, the aborigines lived in relative poverty on a diet consisting mostly of highly refined and denatured food products, a diet deficient in many vital nutrients.

Dr. Kalokerinos determined that many of the aboriginal infants suffered from acute ascorbic acid (vitamin C) deficiency. He postulated that a compromised immune resistance due both to a diet lacking in essential nutrients, especially vitamin C, and to the presence of infectious illness placed many infants in a dangerous state of health. In many children the injection of vaccine, further challenging an already crippled immune system, was sufficient to cause death.

Working on the assumption that these deaths were the result of an interaction of the vaccinations with malnutrition, he instituted an improved nutrition program with regular ascorbic acid supplementation. In addition, he screened infants to avoid giving vaccines during minor illnesses. As a result, infant mortality was virtually abolished. For two years, not one infant under his care died.

Besides diseases of an acute nature, chronic degenerative diseases have also been reported to follow vaccination. Numerous German authors have described the occurrence of multiple sclerosis following administration of vaccines against smallpox, typhoid fever, paratyphoid fever, tetanus, poliomyelitis, tuberculosis, influenza, and rabies.[10] Systemic lupus erythematosis has also been reported to occur after vaccination.[11]

Burton Waisbren posed the following question concerning the apparent immune system-mediated diseases of multiple sclerosis and Guillain-Barré syndrome—notorious due to its tragic occurrence after the ill-fated swine flu vaccine program:

Is it possible that an antigen in the swine-influenza vaccine evokes in some patients an immune response to myelin basic proteins—those that surround the peripheral nerves in patients who developed Guillain-Barré syndrome, and those around the central nerves in patients who developed a disorder similar to multiple sclerosis?[12]

Dr. Robert Couch, Baylor University, Houston, Texas, testified before the United States Public Health Service Immunization Practices Advisory Committee in January 1982 that after flu vaccination of elderly persons who had a history of chronic disorders, six out of seven persons with allergies reported that their allergies became worse; one out of 20 with hypertension noted increased blood pressure; one out of nine with diabetes and two with gout developed a cold, a gout attack, and increased blood sugar; and one on therapy for Parkinson's disease noted increased clumsiness.[13]

In a study of the diphtheria-pertussis-tetanus (DPT) vaccine, only 7 percent of those receiving the vaccine had no untoward reaction; 54 percent had fevers and 82 percent exhibited behavioral changes.[14]

Summary and Conclusions

At the present time an overwhelming majority of the members of the American medical community accept and approve current vaccination programs for children. It should be obvious that this period of early infancy, when children have immature immune systems, is one of extreme vulnerability and susceptibility to vaccinations, especially in the earliest months following birth. Only a handful of physicians and laypersons throughout the decades has objected to these vaccination programs because of suspected adverse side effects. In some instances their arguments have lacked substance, due to the fact that they have sought to demonstrate direct toxicities from the vaccines.

Direct toxicities do occur, but they appear to be relatively uncommon. Most authorities today consider these occasional incidents as an acceptable risk. They believe that the benefits from the vaccines, in terms of control gained over infectious diseases, far outweigh the danger of toxicities.

The real danger appears to be an indirect effect of impairment and malfunction of the immune system. Since this effect is often delayed, indirect, and masked, its true nature is seldom recognized.

In the United States few individuals have braved the wrath of orthodoxy by pointing out the probability of widespread and unrecognized immune system malfunctions that are vaccine-induced, and the need for scientific investigation of these effects. In our opinion there is now sufficient evidence of immune malfunction following current vaccination programs to anticipate a growing public demand for research into alternative methods for prevention of infectious diseases.

The one change that could bring immediate and far-reaching results is to allow absolute freedom of choice in accepting or rejecting vaccines for every individual and every parent. Like the Mississippi River steamboat that is grounded on a sandbar, current research in the prevention of infectious diseases is arrested by the current system of compulsory, mandated vaccination for schoolchildren. If vaccinations are made optional, the situation will become unfrozen. Medical research can then move ahead in search of other workable solutions.

Notes

1. Alexander Schauss, *Diet, Crime, and Delinquency* (Berkeley, CA: Parker House, 1980).
2. Richard Markarness, *Not All in the Mind* (London: Pan Books Ltd., 1980).
3. William H. Phillpott, MD, and Dwight K. Kalita, PhD, *Brain Allergies: The Psychonutrient Connection* (New Canaan, CT: Keats Publishing, Inc., 1980).
4. Theron Randolph, MD, and Ralph Moss, PhD, *An Alternative Approach to Allergies* (New York: Lippincott and Crowell, Publishers, 1979).
5. Marshall Mandell, MD, and Lynne Waller Scanlon, *Dr. Mandell's 5-Day Allergy Relief System* (New York: Thomas Crowell, Publishers, 1979).
6. J. A. Brody and R. McAlister, "Depression of Tuberculin Sensitivity Following Measles Vaccination," *American Review of Respiratory Diseases 90* (1964): 607–611.
7. J. A. Brody, T. Overfield, and L. M. Hammes, "Depression of the Tuberculin Reaction by Viral Vaccines," *New England Journal of Medicine 271* (1964): 1294–1296.
8. Sir Graham Wilson, *The Hazards of Immunization* (New York: Oxford University Press, 1967).
9. Archie Kalokerinos, MD, *Every Second Child* (Melbourne, Australia: Thomas Nelson Limited, 1975).
10. Miller et al., "Multiple Sclerosis and Vaccinations," *British Medical Journal* (22 April 1967): 210–213.
11. L. Fred Ayvazian, MD, "Risks of Repeated Immunization," *Annals of Internal Medicine 82*, no. 4 (April 1975): 589.
12. Burton A. Waisbren, "Swine Influenza Vaccine," *Annals of Internal Medicine 97*, no. 1 (July 1982): 149.
13. Information provided by Dr. Robert Couch, Baylor University, Houston, Texas.
14. R. Barkin et al., "Diphtheria-pertussis-tetanus Vaccine: Reactogenicity of Commercial Products," *Pediatrics 63* (2 February 1979): 256–260.

IMMUNIZATIONS: THE OTHER SIDE

Richard Moskowitz

Richard Moskowitz, MD, received his undergraduate degree from Harvard University and his medical degree from New York University before studying homeopathy with George Vithoulkas in Athens, Greece. He recently served as president of the National Center for Homeopathy in Washington, DC, and is the author of a book on homeopathy in pregnancy and birth to be published in 1993 by North Atlantic Press. A Contributing Editor to Mothering, *Dr. Moskowitz currently practices classical homeopathy in Watertown, Massachusetts. "Immunizations: The Other Side" is an abridged version of an article that originally appeared in the* Journal of the American Institute of Homeopathy *(1983). An earlier version of this article was published in* Mothering, *no. 31 (Spring 1984).*

The growing refusal of parents to vaccinate their children is seldom articulated or taken seriously. The fact is that we have been taught to accept vaccination as a sort of involuntary communion, a sacrament of our own participation in the unrestricted growth of scientific and industrial technology, utterly heedless of the long-term consequences to the health of our own species, not to mention the balance of nature as a whole. For that reason alone, the other side of the case urgently needs to be heard.

Are Vaccines Effective?

There is widespread agreement that we have, in the time period since the common vaccines were introduced, seen a remarkable decline in the incidence and severity of the corresponding natural infections. But the customary assumption that the decline is *attributable* to the vaccines remains unproven, and continues to be seriously questioned by eminent authorities in the field. The incidence and severity of whooping cough had already begun to decline precipitously long before the pertussis vaccine was introduced,[1] a fact which led the epidemiologist C. C. Dauer to remark, as far back as 1943:

If mortality [from pertussis] continues to decline at the same rate during the next 15 years, it will be extremely difficult to show statistically that [pertussis immunization] had any effect in reducing mortality from whooping cough.[2]

Much the same is true not only of diphtheria and tetanus, but also of tuberculosis, cholera, typhoid, and other common scourges of a bygone era, which began to disappear toward the end of the 19th century, perhaps partly in response to improvements in public health and sanitation, but in any case long before antibiotics, vaccines, or any specific medical measures designed to eradicate them.[3]

Reflections such as these led the great microbiologist René Dubos to observe that microbial diseases have their own natural history, independent of drugs and vaccines, in which asymptomatic infection and symbiosis are far more common than overt disease:

It is barely recognized, but nevertheless true, that animals and plants, as well as men, can live peacefully with their most notorious microbial enemies. The world is obsessed by the fact that poliomyelitis can kill and maim several thousand unfortunate victims every year. But more extraordinary is the fact that millions upon millions of young people become infected by polio viruses, yet suffer no harm from the infection. The dramatic episodes of conflict between men and microbes are what strike the mind. What is less readily apprehended is the more common fact that infection can occur without producing disease.[4]

The principal evidence that the vaccines are effective actually dates from the more recent period, during which time the dreaded polio epidemics of the 1940s and 1950s have never reappeared in the developed countries, and measles, mumps, and rubella, which even a generation ago were among the commonest diseases of childhood, have become far less prevalent, at least in their classic acute forms, since the triple MMR vaccine was introduced into common use.

Yet, how the vaccines actually accomplish these changes is not nearly as well understood as most people like to think. The disturbing possibility that they act in some other way than by producing a genuine immunity is suggested by the fact that the diseases in question have continued to break out even in highly immunized populations, and that in such cases the observed differences in incidence and severity between immunized and unimmunized persons have tended to be far less dramatic than expected, and in some cases not measurably significant at all.

In a recent British outbreak of whooping cough, for example, even fully immunized children contracted the disease in fairly large numbers, and the rates of serious complications and death were reduced only slightly.[5] In another recent outbreak of pertussis, 46 of the 85 fully immunized children studied eventually contracted the disease.[6]

In 1977, 34 new cases of measles were reported on the campus of UCLA, in a population that was supposedly 91 percent immune, according to careful serological testing.[7] Another 20 cases of measles were reported in the Pecos, New Mexico, area within a period of a few months in 1981, and at least 75 percent of the people involved had been fully immunized, some quite recently.[8] A survey of sixth graders in a well-immunized urban community revealed that about 15 percent of this group are still susceptible to rubella, a figure essentially identical with that of the prevaccine era.[9]

Finally, although the overall incidence of typical acute measles in the United States has dropped sharply from about 400,000 cases annually in the early 1960s to about 30,000 cases by 1974 to 1976, the death rate has remained exactly the same;[10] and, with the peak incidence now occurring in adolescents and young adults, the risk of pneumonia and demonstrable liver abnormalities has actually increased substantially, according to one recent study, to well over 3 percent and 20 percent, respectively.[11]

The simplest way to explain these discrepancies would be to postulate that the vaccines confer only partial or temporary immunity, which sounds reasonable enough, given the fact that they are either live viruses rendered less virulent by serial passage in tissue culture, or bacteria or bacterial proteins that have been killed or denatured by heat, such that they can still elicit an antibody response but no longer initiate the full-blown disease.

Because the vaccine is a "trick," in the sense that it *stimulates* the true or natural immune response developed in the course of recovering from the actual disease, it is certainly realistic to expect that such artificial immunity will in fact "wear off" quite easily, and even require additional booster doses at regular intervals throughout life to maintain peak effectiveness.

Such an explanation would be disturbing enough for most people. Indeed, the basic fallacy inherent in it is painfully evident in the fact that there is no way to know how long this partial or temporary immunity will last in any given individual, or how often it will need to be restimulated, because the answers to these questions clearly depend on precisely the same individual variables that would have determined whether or how severely the same person, unvaccinated, would have contracted the disease in the first place.

In any case, a number of other observations suggest equally strongly that this simple explanation cannot be the correct one. First, a number of investigators have shown that when a person vaccinated against the measles, for example, again becomes susceptible to it, even repeated booster doses will have little or no effect.[12]

Second, the vaccines do not act merely by producing pale or mild copies of the original disease; all of them also commonly produce a variety of symptoms of their own. Moreover, in some cases, these illnesses may be considerably more serious than the original disease, involving deeper structures, more vital organs, and less of a tendency to resolve spontaneously. Even more worrisome is the fact that they are almost always more difficult to recognize.

Thus, in a recent outbreak of mumps in supposedly immune schoolchildren, several developed atypical symptoms, such as anorexia, vomiting, and erythematous rashes, without any parotid involvement (swollen glands), and the diagnosis required extensive serological testing to rule out other concurrent diseases.[13] The syndrome of "atypical measles" can be equally difficult to diagnose, even when it is thought of,[14] which suggests that it is often overlooked entirely. In some cases, atypical measles can be much more severe than the regular kind, with pneumonia, petechiae, edema, and severe pain,[15] and likewise often goes unsuspected.

In any case, it seems virtually certain that other vaccine-related syndromes will be described and identified, if only we take the trouble to look for them, and that the ones we are aware of so far represent only a very small part of the problem. But even these few make it less and less plausible to assume that the vaccines produce a normal, healthy immunity that lasts for some time but then wears off, leaving the patient miraculously unharmed and unaffected by the experience.

The Individual Vaccines Reconsidered

Next I wish to consider each of the vaccines on an individual basis, in relation to the infectious diseases from which they are derived.

The MMR is composed of attenuated live measles, mumps, and rubella viruses, administered in a single intramuscular injection at about 15 months of age. Subsequent reimmunization is no longer recommended, except for young women of childbearing age, in whom the risk of congenital rubella syndrome (CRS) is thought to warrant it, even though the effectiveness of reimmunization is questionable at best.

Prior to the vaccine era, measles, mumps, and rubella were reckoned among the routine childhood diseases, which most schoolchildren contracted before the age of puberty, and from which nearly all recovered, with permanent, lifelong immunity and with no complications or sequelae.

However, such diseases were not always so harmless. Measles, in particular, can be a devastating disease when a population encounters it *for the first time.* Its importation from Spain, for instance, undoubtedly contributed to Cortez's conquest of the great Aztec empire; whole villages were depopulated by epidemics of measles and smallpox, leaving only a small remnant of cowed, superstitious warriors to face the bearded conquistadors from across the sea.[16] In more recent outbreaks among isolated, primitive peoples, the case fatality rate from measles averaged 20 to 30 percent.[17]

In these so-called virgin-soil epidemics, not only measles but polio and many other similar diseases take their highest toll of death and serious complications among adolescents and young adults—healthy and vigorous people in the prime of life—and leave relatively unharmed the group of children younger than puberty.[18]

This means that the evolution of a disease such as measles from a dreaded killer to an ordinary disease of childhood presupposes the development of nonspecific or "herd" immunity in young children, such that, when they are finally exposed to the disease, it activates defense mechanisms already prepared to receive it, resulting in the long incubation period and the usually benign, self-limited course.

Under these circumstances, the rationale for wanting to vaccinate young children against measles is limited to the fact that a very small number of deaths and serious complications have continued to occur, chiefly pneumonia, encephalitis, and the rare but dreaded subacute sclerosing panencephalitis (SSPE), a slow-virus disease with a reported incidence of 1 per 100,000 cases.[19] Pneumonia, by far the commonest complication, is usually benign and self-limited, even without treatment;[20] and, even in those rare cases in which bacterial pneumonia supervenes, adequate treatment is currently available.

By all accounts, then, the death rate from wild-type measles is very low, the incidence of serious sequelae is insignificant, and the general benefit to the child who recovers from the disease, and to his contacts and descendants, is very great. Consequently, even if the measles vaccine could be shown to reduce the risk of death or serious complications from the disease, it still could not justify the high probability of autoimmune diseases, cancer, and whatever else may result from the propagation of latent measles virus in human tissue culture for life.

The case for immunizing against mumps and rubella seems *a fortiori* even more tenuous, for exactly the same reasons. Mumps is also essentially a benign, self-limited disease in children before the age of puberty, and recovery from a single attack confers lifelong immunity. The principal complication is meningoencephalitis, mild or subclinical forms of which are relatively common, although the death rate is extremely low,[21] and sequelae are rare.

The mumps vaccine is prepared and administered in much the same way as the measles vaccine, usually in the same injection; and the dangers associated with it are likewise comparable. Like measles, mumps is fast becoming a disease of adolescents and young adults,[22] age groups that tolerate the disease much less well. The chief complication is acute epididymoorchitis, which occurs in 30 to 40 percent of the males affected past the age of puberty, and usually results in atrophy of the testicle on the affected side;[23] but it also shows a strong tendency to attack the ovary and the pancreas.

For all of these reasons, the greatest favor we could do for our children would be to expose them all to the measles and mumps when they are young, which would not only protect them against contracting more serious forms of these diseases when they grow older, but would also greatly assist in their immunological maturation with minimal risk. I need hardly add that this is very close to the actual evolution of these diseases before the MMR vaccine was introduced.

The same discrepancy is evident in the case of rubella, or German measles, which in young children is a disease so mild that it frequently escapes detection,[24] but in older children and adults not infrequently produces arthritis, purpura, and other severe, systemic signs.[25] The main impetus for the development of the vaccine was certainly the recognition of the "congenital rubella syndrome (CRS)," resulting from damage to the developing embryo in utero during the first trimester of pregnancy,[26] and the relatively high incidence of CRS traceable to the rubella outbreak of 1964.

But here again, we have an almost entirely benign, self-limited disease transformed by the vaccine into a considerably less benign disease of adolescents and young adults of reproductive age, which is ironically the group that most needs to be protected against it. Moreover, as with measles and mumps, the simplest and most effective way to prevent CRS would be to expose everybody to rubella in elementary school; reinfection does sometimes occur after recovery from rubella, but much less commonly than after vaccination.[27]

The equation looks somewhat different for the diphtheria and tetanus vaccines. First of all, both diphtheria and tetanus are serious, sometimes fatal diseases, even with the best of treatment; this is especially true of tetanus, which still carries a mortality rate of close to 50 percent.

Furthermore, these vaccines are not made from living diphtheria and tetanus organisms, but only from certain toxins elaborated by them. These poisonous substances are still highly antigenic, even after being inactivated by heat. Diphtheria and tetanus toxoids, therefore, do not protect against infections per se, but only against the systemic action of the original poisons, in the absence of which both infections are of minor importance clinically.

Consequently, it is easy to understand why parents might want their children protected against diphtheria and tetanus, if safe and effective protection were available. Moreover, both vaccines have been in use for a long time, and the reported incidence of serious problems has remained very low, so that there has never been much public outcry against them.

On the other hand, both diseases are quite readily controlled by simple sanitary measures and careful attention to wound hygiene; and, in any case, both have been steadily disappearing from the developing countries, since long before the vaccines were introduced.

Diphtheria now occurs sporadically in the United States, often in areas with significant reservoirs of unvaccinated children. But the claim that the vaccine is "protective" is once again belied by the fact that, when the disease does break out, the supposedly "susceptible" children are in fact no more likely to develop clinical diphtheria than their fully immunized contacts. In a 1969 outbreak in Chicago, for example, the Board of Health reported that 25 percent of the cases had been fully immunized, and that another 12 percent had received one or more doses of the vaccine and showed serological evidence of full immunity; another 18 percent had been partly immunized, according to the same criteria.[28]

So, once again we are faced with the probability that what the diphtheria toxoid has produced is not a genuine immunity to diphtheria at all, but rather some sort of chronic immune *tol-*

erance to it, by harboring highly antigenic residues somewhere within the cells of the immune system, presumably with long-term suppressive effects on the immune mechanism generally.

This suspicion is further substantiated by the fact that all of the DPT vaccines are alum-precipitated and preserved with thimerosal, an organomercury derivative, to prevent them from being metabolized too rapidly, so that the antigenic challenge will continue for as long as possible. The fact is that we do not know and have never even attempted to discover what actually becomes of these foreign substances, once they are inside the human body.

Exactly the same problems complicate the record of the tetanus vaccine, which almost certainly has had at least some impact in reducing the incidence of tetanus in its classic acute form, yet presumably also survives for years or even decades as a potent foreign antigen within the body, with long-term incalculable effects on the immune system and elsewhere.

Whooping cough, much like diphtheria and tetanus, began to decline as a serious epidemiological threat long before the vaccine was introduced. Moreover, the vaccine has not been particularly effective, even according to its proponents; and the incidence of known side effects is disturbingly high.

The power of the pertussis vaccine to damage the central nervous system, for example, has received growing attention since Stewart and his colleagues reported an alarmingly high incidence of encephalopathy and severe convulsive disorders in British children that were traceable to the vaccine.[29] My own cases suggest that hematological disturbances may be even more prevalent, and that, in any case, the known complications almost certainly represent a small fraction of the total.

Pertussis is also extremely variable clinically, ranging in severity from asymptomatic, mild, or inapparent infections, which are quite common actually, to very rare cases in young infants less than five months of age, in whom the mortality rate is said to reach 40 percent.[30] Indeed, the disease is rarely fatal or even that serious in children over one year of age, and antibiotics have very little to do with the outcome.[31]

A good deal of the pressure to immunize at the present time thus seems to be attributable to the higher death rate in very young infants, which has led to the terrifying practice of giving this most clearly dangerous of the vaccines to infants at two months of age, when their mothers' milk would normally protect them from all infections about as well as can ever be done,[32] and when the effect on the still developing blood and nervous systems could be catastrophic.

Poliomyelitis and the polio vaccines present an entirely different situation. The standard Sabin vaccine is trivalent, consisting of attenuated, live polioviruses of each of the three strains associated with poliomyelitis; but it is administered orally, in much the same way as the infection is acquired in nature. The oral or noninjectable route, which leaves the recipient free to develop a natural immunity at the normal portal of entry, that is, the GI tract, would therefore appear to represent a considerable safety factor.

On the other hand, the wild-type poliovirus produces no symptoms whatsoever in over 90 percent of the people who contract it, even under epidemic conditions;[33] and, of those people who do come down with recognizable clinical disease, perhaps only 1 or 2 percent ever progress to the full-blown neurological picture of poliomyelitis, with its characteristic lesions in the anterior horn cells of the spinal cord or medulla oblongata.[34]

Poliomyelitis thus presupposes peculiar conditions of susceptibility in the host, even a specific *anatomical* susceptibility, since, even under epidemic conditions, the virulence of the poliovirus is so low, and the number of cases resulting in death or permanent disability is always remarkably small.[35]

Given the fact that the poliovirus was ubiquitous before the vaccine was introduced, and could be found routinely in samples of city sewage wherever it was looked for,[36] it is evident that effective, natural immunity to poliovirus was already as close to being universal as it can ever be, and *a fortiori* no artificial substitute could ever equal or even approximate that result. Indeed, because the virulence of the poliovirus was so low to begin with, it is difficult to see what further attenuation of it could possibly accomplish, other than to abate as well the full vigor of the natural immune response to it.

For the fact remains that even the attenuated virus is still alive, and the people who were anatomically susceptible to it before are still susceptible to it now. This means, of course, that at least *some* of these same people will develop paralytic polio from the vaccine,[37] and that the others may still be harboring the virus in latent form, perhaps within those same cells.

The only obvious advantage of giving the vaccine, then, would be to introduce people to the virus when they are still infants, at a time when the virulence is normally lowest anyway;[38] but even this benefit could be more than offset by the danger of weakening the immune response. In any case, the whole matter is clearly one of enormous complexity, and illustrates only too well the hidden dangers and miscalculations that are inherent in the virtually irresistible attempt to beat nature at her own game, to eliminate a problem that cannot be eliminated, namely the susceptibility to disease itself.

Even in the case of the polio vaccine, then, which appears to be about as safe as any vaccine ever *can* be, the same fundamental dilemma remains. Perhaps the day will come when we can face the consequences of deliberately feeding live polioviruses to every living infant, and admit that we should have left well enough alone and addressed ourselves to the art of healing the sick rather than to the technology of eradicating the *possibility* of sickness, when we do not have to, and cannot possibly succeed in any case.

Notes

1. E. Mortimer, "Pertussis Immunization," *Hospital Practice* (October 1980): 103.
2. Quoted in ibid., p. 105.
3. René Dubos, *The Mirage of Health* (New York: Harper & Row, 1959), p. 73.
4. Ibid., pp. 74–75.
5. G. Stewart, "Vaccination against Whooping Cough: Efficiency vs. Risks," *The Lancet* (1977): 234.
6. *Medical Tribune* (10 January 1979): 1.
7. J. Cherry, "The New Epidemiology of Measles and Rubella," *Hospital Practice* (July 1980): 52–54.
8. Unpublished data from the New Mexico Health Department (private communication).
9. M. Lawless et al., "Rubella Susceptibility in Sixth-Graders," *Pediatrics 65* (June 1980): 1086–1089.
10. See Note 7, p. 49.
11. *Infectious Diseases* (January 1982): 21.
12. See Note 7, p. 52.
13. *Family Practice News* (15 July 1980): 1.

14. J. Ferrante, "Atypical Symptoms? It Could *Still* Be Measles," *Modern Medicine* (30 September 1980): 76.

15. See Note 7, p. 53.

16. W. McNeill, *Plagues and Peoples* (New York: Doubleday, 1976), p. 184.

17. M. Burnet and D. White, *The Natural History of Infectious Disease* (Cambridge, MA: Harvard University Press, 1972), p. 16.

18. Ibid., pp. 90, 121.

19. A. Steigman, "Slow Virus Infections," in Victor Vaughan and R. J. McKay, *Nelson Textbook of Pediatrics,* 11th ed. (Philadelphia: W. B. Saunders, Co., 1979), p. 937.

20. C. Phillips, in Vaughan et al., *Nelson Textbook of Pediatrics,* p. 860.

21. C. Phillips, "Mumps," in Vaughan et al., *Nelson Textbook of Pediatrics,* p. 891.

22. G. Hayden et al., "Mumps and Mumps Vaccine in the U.S.," *Continuing Education* (September 1979): 97.

23. See Note 21, p. 892.

24. C. Phillips, "Rubella," in Vaughan et al., *Nelson Textbook of Pediatrics,* p. 863.

25. Ibid., p. 862.

26. L. Glasgow and J. Overall, "Congenital Rubella Syndrome," in Vaughan et al., *Nelson Textbook of Pediatrics,* p. 483.

27. See Note 24, p. 865.

28. Cited in R. Mendelsohn, "The Truth about Immunizations," *The People's Doctor* (April 1978): 1.

29. See Note 5, p. 234.

30. R. Feigin, "Pertussis," in Vaughan et al., *Nelson Textbook of Pediatrics,* p. 769.

31. Ibid.

32. L. Barness, "Breast Feeding," in Vaughan et al., *Nelson Textbook of Pediatrics,* p. 191.

33. See Note 17, pp. 91ff.

34. B. Davis et al., *Microbiology,* 2nd ed. (New York: Harper & Row, 1973), pp. 1290ff.

35. Ibid., p. 1280.

36. See Note 17, p. 93.

37. V. Fulginiti, "Problems of Poliovirus Immunization," *Hospital Practice* (August 1980): 61–62.

38. See Note 17, p. 95.

BRINGING VACCINES INTO PERSPECTIVE

Harold E. Buttram and John Chriss Hoffman

Harold E. Buttram, MD, is a general practitioner in addition to specializing in allergy and environmental medicine. He lives in Quakertown, Pennsylvania. John Chriss Hoffman studied for his PhD in microbiology at the Catholic University in Washington, DC, and has been involved in the vaccination debate since 1978. "Bringing Vaccines into Perspective" first appeared in Mothering, *no. 34 (Winter 1985).*

At present there are two schools of thought concerning state and federally enforced vaccine programs for children and infants. On the one hand, an overwhelming majority of the members of the American medical and public health communities approve current vaccination programs; they accept the occasional toxic vaccine reaction in children as the price that must be paid for the seeming control gained over infectious diseases.

On the other hand, a small but growing minority of physicians and laypersons express concern about these vaccine programs, believing that the harm done from them may be far more extensive than generally recognized. All too often, the arguments of this latter group have lacked credibility because of a deficiency of concrete scientific evidence. In our opinion, this is now changing.

Increase in Allergic (Atopic) Disorders

Many practicing physicians in the United States and Europe have made the observation that allergic and/or immunologic disorders in children are rapidly increasing. In a review in *Modern Medicine* (May 1983) of an international allergy meeting in London, it was stated: "There is little doubt that the incidence of allergic disorders has increased in recent years."[1] One prominent pediatrician has speculated that "there may be a relationship between immunization as a stress and the onset of some of the devastating array of symptoms I am seeing all the time in younger and younger children."[2]

In a survey conducted by Eaton[3] the incidence of allergic problems in a sample population of women in England increased from 25 percent in 1974 to 32 percent in 1979; in men, reported allergic problems increased from 20 percent in 1974 to 27 percent in 1979. This represents an increased incidence of allergies of over 1 percent per year for the population surveyed. Atherton reported an alarming increase in atopic eczema in Great Britain.[4] Of a group of 12,555 children born in a single week in 1970, 12 percent were reported by their parents to have had atopic eczema by the age of five years,[5] more than twice the proportion reported in a similar study 12 years previously.

From our point of view, there may be several major factors in modern society that can potentially cause an immunologic weakening of our children. Such causes may include chemical pollution of air, food, and water; commercial formula feeding, instead of breastfeeding; excessive use of drugs in children and in mothers during pregnancy and lactation; and commercial food processing and devitalization.[6] In addition, current mass vaccination programs must be highly suspected as contributing to the increased incidence of allergic disorders.

Lymphocyte Abnormality Following
Tetanus Booster Shots

A significant report appeared in the correspondence section of *The New England Journal of Medicine* (19 January 1984) entitled "Abnormal T-Lymphocyte Subpopulations in Healthy Subjects after Tetanus Booster Immunization."[7] The letter reported studies conducted to determine the effects of booster vaccination with tetanus toxoid on the ratio of the helper-to-suppressor T-lymphocytes of healthy adults. Indirect immunofluorescence evaluation of T-lymphocytes from blood samples taken before and after booster vaccination revealed a temporary drop, for each subject, in the helper/suppressor ratio after vaccination. The largest drop detected occurred between days 3 and 14 postvaccination, with 4 of the 11 subjects demonstrating ratios of 1.0 or less (normal values are in the range of 1.0 to 2.0). *The report pointed out that similar drops in helper/suppressor ratios of T-lymphocytes are characteristic of Acquired Immune Deficiency Syndrome (AIDS).*

The question is: Does a similar AIDS-like state occur in young children and infants following their receipt of multiple-vaccine regimens during the crucial period of their lives when their immune system is beginning to mature? Any suppression of the helper T-lymphocytes during this time, even of a transient nature, would most certainly be undesirable. What is known is that an AIDS-like reduced T-lymphocyte ratio has been described in *young children* and may be the underlying cause of transient hypogammaglobulinemia (reduced level of protective immunoglobulins in the blood) in *infancy.*[8] As yet unresolved is the role that vaccines given in infancy play in producing this immunologic disorder. However, for many years immunologists have been aware of a state of anergy (immunologic unresponsiveness) following vaccination. J. A. Brody and others reported that live-virus vaccines have been shown to transiently suppress tuberculin sensitivity.[9,10]

As reviewed in the booklet *The Dangers of Immunization,*[11] a partial list of vaccine-related diseases and/or immunologic disorders reported in the medical literature would include the following: Sudden Infant Death Syndrome (SIDS), Guillain-Barré syndrome, lupus erythematosus, multiple sclerosis, arthritis (in adults following rubella vaccine), and worsening of allergies (in elderly persons following influenza vaccinations).

One of the most extensively documented reports of the indirect effects of vaccines is found in the book *The Hazards of Immunization*[12] by Sir Graham Wilson, formerly of the Public Health Laboratory Service, England and Wales. Although Dr. Wilson was not generally opposed to vaccines, he provided a number of documented historical examples in which vaccination against one disease seemed to provoke another.

The first full recognition and description in modern times of immune malfunction following vaccinations should be ascribed to two Australians, Archie Kalokerinos, MD, and Glen Dettman, PhD, as reported in the book *Every Second Child*.[13] In this book Dr. Kalokerinos describes his work as a physician in the 1960s and 1970s among Australian aborigines. In early work with these people, he was appalled by the high infant mortality rate; death rates in some areas had soared to 50 percent.

The Australian aborigines were a unique population. They lacked the natural resistance to many infectious diseases to which Western civilization has been exposed throughout the centuries. Also, the aborigines lived in relative poverty on a diet consisting mostly of highly refined and denatured food products.

Dr. Kalokerinos (later joined by Dr. Dettman) determined that many of the aboriginal infants suffered from acute ascorbic acid (vitamin C) deficiency. He postulated that a compromised immune resistance, due both to a diet lacking in essential nutrients (especially vitamin C) and to the presence of infectious illness, placed many infants in a high-risk state. In many children, the injection of vaccine further challenged an already crippled immune system and was enough to bring on death.

The present report, showing lymphocyte abnormality with AIDS-like changes following tetanus vaccine, provides a theoretical explanation for these deaths. It may also provide a partial explanation for the known increase in allergic disorders in our own contemporary population.

Mucosal Vaccinations

If vaccinations are to be used to attempt to control infectious diseases, both intuition and reason should compel us to seek those methods that most closely simulate natural immunity, methods which can be utilized without crippling the immune system of the body.

Today, there is increasing interest in and investigation of the mucosal vaccines, of which oral (Sabin) poliovirus vaccine may be considered an example. However, oral poliovirus vaccines, which consist of live viruses grown in animal tissue cultures, are administered in large numbers. Vaccination with these live viruses can and does cause problems.

The subject of mucosal vaccines was reviewed by P. L. Ogra in 1980, and by John Bienenstock in 1983.[14, 15] In contrast to injected vaccines, which bypass the outer defenses of the body, mucosal vaccines more closely follow the processes of natural immunity. Why is this so?

There are five known classes of immunoglobulins (antibodies which serve as immunologic defenses) in the body: IgM, IgG, IgA, IgE, and IgD. The IgC (gamma globulin) antibodies form the largest quantity in the bloodstream, along with IgM (macroglobulins). In contrast, the IgA (secretory immunoglobulin A) antibodies coat the mucosal surfaces of the body, including the gastrointestinal, respiratory, and genitourinary tracts, where they function as "antiseptic paint."[16, 17, 18] From a conceptual standpoint, the IgA antibodies form the first line of immunologic defense of the body, whereas the IgG and IgM antibodies form the last line of antibody defense.

It is clearly evident that most infectious diseases find their way into the body through the mucosal surfaces (lungs, gastrointestinal tract, and so forth). Consequently, "natural immunity" is largely a mucosal immunity involving the secretory immunoglobulin A(IgA) antibodies. Current research appears to support this concept.[19, 20]

Modern vaccines, with the exception (to some degree) of the oral poliovirus vaccine, are contrary to the principles of natural immunity. They are injected into the body, where they stimulate IgG antibodies (last line of antibody defense) rather than IgA antibodies (first line of immunologic defense).

This concept is borne out experimentally. In a comparison of injected, killed poliovirus vaccine with live, attenuated oral poliovirus vaccine, only the oral vaccine produced protective secretory immunoglobulin (IgA) antibodies against polio on the mucosal surfaces of the body.[21]

We would like to see our country be in the vanguard of vaccine research, but we are relatively stagnant in this area, with investigations largely limited to the unphysiologic, injected vaccines. Other countries, in contrast, appear to be making significant advances in new dimensions of vaccine research. Writing in *Fortschritte der Medizin*, Falk at the University of Graz in Vienna described the administration of oral pertussis (whooping cough) vaccine to 13,770 newborn infants in 1978, 1979,

and 1980 in two pediatric hospitals in Austria.[22] It was reported that oral pertussis vaccine lowered the risk of side effects because
toxic components were not taken up by receptors in the infants'
gastrointestinal tracts. The oral vaccine was tolerated well. The
vaccine could be given within the infant's first few days of life,
providing the beginning of protection at the strategic time
when the child may be at greatest risk. That it appeared to provide both local and general immunity may be another plus.

Present understanding of the total impact of vaccine programs on the immune system is virtually nonexistent. Until
more is known, we believe that the oral (mucosal) vaccines are
closer to the processes of natural immunity and, therefore, presumably safer than injected vaccines. We can only ask why we are
not pursuing this line of investigation more aggressively.

Inapparent Infections and Natural Immunity

For those who are honestly trying to weigh the pros and cons
of vaccines, one fundamental question arises: What are the
basic differences between natural immunity and vaccines? Each
time we scratch our skin we are inoculated with bacteria. When
we inhale cold or flu viruses from a sick person, we experience
a form of immunization. We may ask ourselves what can be the
harm from vaccines when we are exposed to potentially infectious agents many times in the course of an ordinary day in our
lives? This question is easily answered. A little analysis, based on
scientific findings, will reveal that there are fundamental, perhaps irreconcilable differences between current methods of vaccination and natural immunity.

The first difference is the *quantity* of antigenic stimulation in modern vaccines. In the case of natural immunity, it has been estimated that the frequency of unnoticed infections outnumber clinical illnesses by at least one hundredfold.[23] Evidence for this is substantiated by the high proportion of adults who have virus-neutralizing substances in their blood serum and the number who, during an epidemic, excrete virus without being ill.

If the immune system is maintained "battle ready" by healthful living, adequate rest, sanitation, and simple and wholesome nutrition, then many diseases will pass as subclinical infections without actual illness, or if there is illness, it will be relatively mild. Under these circumstances, we may assume that small amounts of antigenic (infectious) material break through the outer defenses. This limited penetration is probably sufficient to produce an immune response but not to cause illness or to overwhelm the immune system. *Nature heals "homeopathically" (by small doses). Natural immunity is probably based on the same principle.*

The first difference, then, between current childhood vaccines and natural immunity is in the *quantity* of antigenic material. In the former there is the introduction of massive quantities of antigen into the system; in the latter the quantities are small. The second major difference, as outlined in the previous section, is in the route of introduction into the system. Most unnoticed infections enter through the mucosal surfaces of the body (respiratory tract, gastrointestinal tract, and so forth) and result in mucosal immunity. Most modern vaccines, on the other hand, are injected directly into the bloodstream.

If we are to search for methods of vaccination which more close-

ly simulate the processes of natural immunity, it would appear
that we are reduced to one area, that of *mucosal vaccines given
in small doses.*

This brings us to the next question. Has there been any
research involving this method of vaccination? We are aware of
one attempt to study homeopathic smallpox vaccine a number
of years ago among a small group of homeopaths, the results
of which were never published.[24] Beyond this, we know of none.

We believe there is a great wealth of scientific talent in this
country that should be directed toward investigation of mucosal vaccines, in very small doses. In our opinion, there is no area
of scientific investigation with greater possibilities and greater
need.

The One Cell, One Antibody Rule

In the healthy person, natural immunity is based on a series
of body defenses, much as the defenses of a medieval fortified
castle. According to this conceptual model, each level of
immunologic defense against invading viruses, bacteria, and so
forth acts as a shock absorber, so that the impact of invading
microorganisms on the bloodstream may be greatly reduced.
In contrast to this principle, most current inoculations inject
massive amounts of vaccine directly into the bloodstream, thus
bypassing the outer defenses of the body.

By way of illustration, let us assume that a child is born with
a total immune capacity of 100 units. According to the *one cell,
one antibody* rule, once an immune body (plasma cell or lymphocyte)
becomes committed to a given antigen, it becomes incapable
of responding to other antigens or challenges.[25, 26, 27] Let us assume

that 25 years ago this hypothetical child passed through the so-called usual childhood diseases of former decades (measles, mumps, chicken pox, and so on) with relatively minor and uncomplicated illnesses. Considering the extreme efficiency of natural immunity, we may make an educated guess that permanent immunity to these diseases was gained by utilizing only 3 to 7 percent of the total immune capacity. In the case of the routine childhood vaccines, however, it is likely that a higher percentage becomes committed, perhaps somewhere from 30 to 70 percent. It should be emphasized that *once an immune body becomes committed to a specific antigen, it becomes inert and incapable of responding to other challenges.*

While this concept is largely hypothetical at this time, it is compatible with our present understanding of the immune system. As reviewed in current texts dealing with pediatrics and immunology,[28, 29, 30, 31] the human newborn infant comes into the world with a relatively undeveloped immune system. The lymph nodes are small, the plasma cells are sparse in the bone marrow and lymph nodes, and immunoglobulin synthesis is low. Normally, soon after birth, the infant begins to respond to multiple antigenic stimuli from the bacterial florae that rapidly populate his or her skin, respiratory tract, and bowel, as well as microbial and parasitic infections (estimated at one every six weeks until age 12) acquired from the environment.

If the immunologic system is normal, this immunologic experience is reflected in progressive hyperplasia of the lymph follicles and the appearance of plasma cells in lymphoid tissues and bone marrow. Also, there is a gradual increase in immunoglobulin synthesis, with gradually rising blood serum levels until approximately six years of age.

According to this model, the immature system of a newborn infant depends on antigenic stimulation for its development. In this sense, *exposure of the infant to viral and bacterial microorganisms may be necessary for normal development of the immune system,* if such exposures come about in a natural manner. When antigenic stimulation comes about in the form of natural environmental challenges, which filter through a series of natural body defenses, then the immune system is developed, strengthened, and matured in the process. If, on the other hand, the immature immune system is compelled to respond to a series of immunizations which bypass the outer defenses, and inject massive antigenic material directly into the body, then the inner immune defense system must divert a large portion of its resources and reserves in responding to this immunologic "shock treatment."

The combined effects of massive, repeated antigenic stimulation from vaccines, which short-circuit the processes of natural immunity and which are given at an extremely vulnerable time of life, cannot help but have adverse effects on the immunologic system of the child, possibly leaving this system crippled in its ability to protect the child throughout life.

In addressing the issues involved in current childhood vaccines (which include tetanus, diphtheria, pertussis, polio, mumps, measles, and rubella), there are some uncertainties that should be acknowledged. First, these vaccines can provide protection from the illness caused by their respective infectious agent, but the percentage of children who will be protected by these vaccines varies with each vaccine. For example, the poliovirus vaccine provides a high percentage of protection, whereas the pertussis vaccine provides a low to moderate percentage. Also, the length of time that the protection persists varies with different vaccines. The protection may be of relatively short duration, as with tetanus toxoid, or simply unknown, as with measles, rubella, mumps, and polio vaccines.

It is not known what would happen if current vaccine programs were stopped or substantially reduced. No one would accept a return to the epidemics of former eras when polio, diphtheria, smallpox, and whooping cough (the so-called killer diseases) decimated childhood populations. Yet, we do not know the extent of the damage, either from direct toxicities or immune malfunction, resulting from the use of vaccines. Does the use of vaccines, with their adverse effects, remain the price that must be paid for control over infectious diseases? Or are the vaccines themselves a scourge, having replaced the diseases they were meant to prevent?

This brings us to the most important question: Are vaccines the only alternative for disease prevention? Much of the success over these killer diseases, ordinarily attributed to the vaccines, has been due to improved general health and sanitation. Nearly 90 percent of the total decline in the death rate of children due to whooping cough, diphtheria, and measles between 1850 and 1940 occurred *before* the introduction of antibiotics and widespread immunizations.[32]

As further evidence that sanitation, rather than vaccinations, has played *the* major role in control of the killer diseases (with the possible exception of polio), we offer the example of smallpox. Most people probably credit the smallpox vaccine with playing the major role in recent eradication of smallpox throughout the world, but let us examine the facts. In the article "Vaccines: A Therapy in Question,"[33] statistics show that less than 10 percent of children in developing countries have received vaccines. With less than 10 percent vaccination participation, mass vaccination programs clearly played no part in smallpox eradication in developing countries. Quite possibly, selective smallpox vaccination in conjunction with quarantine measures did play an important part in the protection of those who might be exposed to smallpox, but mass smallpox vaccination was not necessary for the eradication of smallpox.

There is a strong and growing body of evidence which suggests that vaccine programs may be weakening the immune systems of our children and thus may be opening the way for other diseases as a result of immunologic dysfunction.

What can be done? While sanitation and improved general health must remain the keystones for control of infectious diseases, there is urgent need for new emphasis on medical research. If vaccines are to be used, methods should be sought which are more in keeping with the processes of natural immunity.

Since the problem is partly political in nature, we believe that major changes in this situation will not come about as long as vaccine programs remain compulsory. If parents are allowed free choice in accepting or rejecting the vaccines for their children, research will be compelled to move ahead, to the ultimate benefit and welfare of our children. In support of this position, we simply point out that vaccines remain voluntary and *noncompulsory* in England, Ireland, West Germany, Austria, Spain, the Netherlands, and Switzerland. We should follow these examples. In a free society such as America, there should be inherent checks and balances in order to allow free choice to the individual in matters that concern his or her personal welfare. Nothing else works quite as well.

Notes

1. Editorial, *Modern Medicine* (May 1983): 57–62.
2. Personal communication.
3. K. K. Eaton, "Incidence of Allergy—Has It Changed?" *Clinical Allergy 12* (1982): 107–110.
4. D. J. Atherton, "Breastfeeding and Atopic Eczema," *British Medical Journal 287* (17 September 1983): 775–776.
5. N. R. Butler and J. Golding, eds., *From Birth to Five: A Study of the Health and Behaviour of Britain's Five Year Olds* (New York: Pergamon, 1986).
6. Harold E. Buttram, *The Dangers of Immunization* (Quakertown, PA: The Humanitarian Society, 1983), pp. 27–28.
7. Martha Eibl et al., "Abnormal T-Lymphocyte Subpopulations in Healthy Subjects after Tetanus Booster Immunization," *New England Journal of Medicine 310*, no. 3 (19 January 1984): 1307–1313.
8. R. L. Siegel, Thomas Issekutz, Jerold Schwaber, Fred Rosen, and Raif Geha, "Deficiency of T-Helper Cells in Transient Hypogammaglobulinemia of Infancy," *New England Journal of Medicine 305*, no. 22 (26 November 1981): 1307–1313.
9. J. A. Brody and R. McAlister, "Depression of Tuberculin Sensitivity Following Measles Vaccination," *American Review of Respiratory Diseases 90* (1964): 607–611.
10. J. A. Brody, T. Overfield, and L. M. Hammes, "Depression of the Tuberculin Reaction by Viral Vaccines," *New England Journal of Medicine 271* (1964): 1294–1296.
11. See Note 6, pp. 9–15.
12. Graham Wilson, *The Hazards of Immunization* (New York: Oxford University Press, 1967).
13. Archie Kalokerinos, MD, *Every Second Child* (Melbourne, Australia: Thomas Nelson Limited, 1974). Available from Thomas Nelson Limited, 597 Little Collins St., Melbourne 3000, Australia.
14. P. L. Ogra, "Viral Vaccination Via the Mucosal Routes," *Review of Infectious Diseases 2*, no. 3 (May/June 1980): 352–369.
15. J. Bienenstock et al. ,"Regulation of Lymphoblast Traffic and Localization in Mucosal Tissues, with Emphasis on IgA," *Federation Proceedings 42*, no. 15 (December 1983): 3213–3217.
16. W. A. Walker, "Antigen Absorption from the Small Intestine and Gas-

trointestinal Disease," *Pediatric Clinics of North America 22,* no. 4 (November 1975): 713–746.

17. W. A. Walker and Richard Hong, "Immunology of the Gastrointestinal Tract," *Journal of Pediatrics 83,* no. 4 (October 1973): 517–530.

18. W. A. Walker et al., "Intestinal Uptake of Macromolecules: Studies on the Mechanism by Which Immunization Interferes with Antigen Uptake," *Journal of Immunology 115* (September 1975): 854–861.

19. See Note 14.

20. See Note 15.

21. See Note 14.

22. W. Falk et al., "The Present and Future of Oral Pertussis Vaccination," *Fortschritte der Medizin* (10 September 1981): 1363–1366.

23. *Maxcy-Rosenaw Preventive Medicine and Public Health,* 10th ed. (New York: Appleton-Century-Crofts, 1973), p. 117.

24. Harold E. Buttram and John Chriss Hoffman, *Vaccination and Immune Malfunction* (Quakertown, PA: Humanitarian Society, 1983), pp. 44–45.

25. F. M. Burnet, *The Clonal Selection Theory of Acquired Immunity* (New York: Cambridge University Press, 1959).

26. R. W. Dutton et al., "Cell Populations and Cell Proliferation in the In Vitro Response of Normal Mouse Spleen to Heterologous Erythrocytes, Etc.," *Journal of Experimental Medicine 126* (1967): 443.

27. Elliott Middleton, Charles Reed, and Elliot Ellis, *Allergy: Principles and Practice* (St. Louis, MO: C. V. Mosby Company, 1983), pp. 3–4.

28. Victor Vaughan and R. J. McKay, *Nelson Textbook of Pediatrics* (Philadelphia: W. B. Saunders, Co., 1975), pp. 474–480.

29. C. W. Bierman and David S. Pearlman, *Allergic Diseases of Infancy, Childhood, and Adolescence* (Philadelphia: W. B. Saunders, Co., 1980), pp. 27–35.

30. Richard E. Stiehm and Vincent A. Fulginiti, *Immunologic Disorders of Infants and Children* (Philadelphia: W. B. Saunders, Co., 1980), pp. 36–51.

31. Joseph A. Bellanti, *Immunology II* (Philadelphia: W. B. Saunders, Co., 1978), pp. 65–77.

32. Statistics presented at the presidential address of the British Association for the Advancement of Sciences by Porter, 1971.

33. "Vaccines: A Therapy in Question," *Therapoeia!* (June 1981): 23.

DPT: A SHOT IN THE DARK

DPT: A Shot in the Dark
Harris L. Coulter and Barbara Loe
   Fisher
Harcourt Brace Jovanovich, 1985

DPT: A Shot in the Dark, by Harris L. Coulter and Barbara Loe Fisher, is a compilation of information about a very controversial subject: the mass, mandatory use of the pertussis vaccine in the United States.

The book is a monumental work of documentation concerning various aspects of pertussis (whooping cough) and pertussis immunization. It provides a comprehensive history of the disease, beginning with reports from the 17th century and continuing with a discussion of the disease in various developed and undeveloped countries today. In addition, this book reviews the original research involved in the development of the pertussis vaccine, its present status, possible side effects, contraindications to its use, and the present efforts to find a safer vaccine. Various political and economic factors involved in use of the vaccine are also discussed.

The major message of the book can be found in the following points:

■ Although pertussis was a highly virulent disease in earlier centuries with high incidence of death as well as non-fatal complications, current evidence indicates that whooping cough has become a milder disease in developed nations with good nutrition, medical care, and sanitation. The United States witnessed a steady drop in whooping cough deaths from the end of the 19th century until the 1930s. This decrease in death rate occurred *before* the widespread use of the pertussis vaccine.

The authors stress that in undeveloped countries, in contrast to developed countries, pertussis remains a virulent disease with death rates of up to 25 percent.

■ Today, the whole-cell pertussis vaccine is made in essentially the same way as in the early 1900s when first developed by Bordet and Bengou. Tests for its safety have been frought with difficulty and remain incomplete. No large clinical trials of any kind have ever been conducted in the United States to measure the vaccine's safety. Serious complications from the vaccine reported in the medical literature include convulsions, hyperkinesis, mental retardation, and death. Although severe complications have been thought to be relatively rare, there has been no mandatory system requiring physicians to report observed complications, and it is possible that the actual incidence of complications may be far greater than previously recognized.

■ According to statistics from England and West Germany, where less than one-third of children are given the pertussis vaccine, the incidence of pertussis in those countries is several times that in the United States, where over 90 percent of children are vaccinated. Nevertheless, the death rates in

England and West Germany from the disease remain very low.

Extrapolating from the reported incidence of whooping cough and its complications in England and West Germany, and from recent studies in the United States concerning possible complications from the vaccine, it is possible that the harm from the vaccine outweighs its benefits. In other words, the complications from the vaccine may be greater than from the disease, in its present mild form in the developed countries of the world.

■ Above all, the authors stress freedom of choice for parents in accepting or rejecting the vaccine for their children. They also stress the great need to pursue the search for a safer vaccine.

This book cannot help but have an effect on complacency concerning the pertussis vaccine and on stimulating a fundamental reevaluation of its currently mandated use in infants and children.

Harold E. Buttram, MD

Harold E. Buttram, MD, is a general practitioner in addition to specializing in allergy and environmental medicine. He lives in Quakertown, Pennsylvania.

VACCINATIONS AND INDIVIDUAL FREEDOM

Vicki Giles

"Vaccinations and Individual Freedom" first appeared in Mothering, *no. 39 (Spring 1986).*

There can be no doubt that any medicine which is potent enough to be effective has at least some potential for toxicity as well. Parents should be aware of the following precautions when dealing with routine vaccinations:

■ *Do not allow your child to be immunized if he or she has been ill or has had a cold or runny nose within the last 48 hours.* Vaccinations provide immunity by going directly into the bloodstream, and an immune system that is already taxed is more likely to react badly to immunization. Vaccinations also affect the lymphatic system, which may already be stressed by a cold or runny nose.

■ *If you wish to have your child vaccinated, consider beginning at six months rather than six weeks. If your child was small for gestational age or was born prematurely, consider waiting even longer.* Although most physicians would recommend that immunizations be started at six weeks because the risk of pertussis, for example, is greater in infancy, there have never been any controlled studies done to determine whether or not an infant under six months of age can actually build immunity when immunized. Booster shots became popular to protect against the possibility that early immunity may not develop through immunization.

In Great Britain, vaccinations are started at six months of age. Why do we start them so much sooner in the United States? The major reasoning for beginning vaccinations so early comes from a study conducted by Parke-Davis in 1962, which concluded that it is more likely that children will receive the entire series of vaccinations if they are begun early in infancy. And, since most babies visit the doctor at four to six weeks for a checkup, it is more convenient for the health practitioner to start the series of immunizations at this time.

■ *If you have a family history of central nervous system disease, deafness, blindness, convulsions, or life-threatening allergies, the pertussis vaccine may be contraindicated for your child.* The pertussis part of the DPT vaccine is considered quite crude. The "whole-cell" pertussis vaccine given to American children has not been separated; the child receives the part of the pertussis cell that generates immunity to the disease along with the part that causes toxic reactions. Current research may be able to isolate the toxic element.

■ *If one child in your family has had a serious reaction to the pertussis vaccine, the child's siblings should probably not receive the vaccine.* Children in the same family tend to react similarly to the pertussis vaccine. The reason for this is not clear.

■ *If your child has exhibited a severe reaction to the pertussis vaccine, immediately find a physician who will verify the reaction and write in your child's permanent medical record that he or she should never again receive a pertussis shot.*

Once a particular child has reacted seriously, additional doses will frequently cause more serious reactions. A serious reaction to vaccination may include any of the following: excessive, high-pitched screaming (the high-pitched scream is suggestive of central nervous system irritation); severe swelling or redness at the site of the injection; fever lasting several days; collapse or extreme lethargy; grayish skin color and cool extremities; or convulsions.

If your child exhibits any of these symptoms, be sure to notify your health professionals and urge them to report the reaction to the federal Centers for Disease Control (CDC), Atlanta, along with the lot and batch number of the vaccination given. Some physicians might not consider local swelling and fever lasting several days to be severe reactions; but there have been cases of children who have exhibited swelling and fever reactions to a first immunization and more severe reactions to a second one, so even swelling and fever should not be discounted.

Some practitioners suggest a half dose followed by another half dose for children who have exhibited a toxic reaction to the vaccine. However, all available evidence indicates that giving the child a half dose of DPT, followed one week later by another half dose, does *not* lessen the potential for toxic reaction.

■ *Always write down the batch and lot number of any vaccine that your child is given.* Be sure to look carefully at the vial whenever your child is given a vaccination. It is possible for a person to make a mistake and give your child the wrong vaccine.

If for any reason your child becomes ill enough to be hospitalized within two weeks following a vaccination, fully describe the course of illness to the health center where the child was given the vaccination. Urge the healthcare professionals to report the reaction and the batch and lot number to the CDC. This will help the CDC statistically analyze whether the batch is particularly reactive or whether your child is overly sensitive to vaccination.

Many, perhaps most, doctors do not consistently report adverse reactions to vaccines. Consequently, the CDC lacks clinical figures for how often a particular vaccine is reactive.

■ *For about two weeks after receiving the "live" polio vaccine, keep your child away from anyone who is not fully immunized against polio, anyone who has an immune deficiency (for example, Acquired Immune Deficiency Syndrome or a deficiency due to chemotherapy) for their own protection.*

The "live" polio vaccine, a live virus, is contagious. Because the disease is carried in the bodily excretions, it is especially important to refuse to allow people who have an immune deficiency to change your baby's diapers.

Be aware that most doctors recommend not giving your child aspirin following the live polio vaccine, because aspirin use has been associated with Reye's syndrome when a child is ill with a virus. A "killed" polio vaccine is also available, but it is not thought to be as effective as the live vaccine.

The concept of "herd immunity" is based on the belief that if *most* people in a community are immune to a disease, an epidemic can be prevented. However, those in favor of 100 percent vaccination do not seem to recognize the fact that not *everyone* who receives a vaccine for a particular disease will be totally immune to this disease. The belief that allowing one person to be free from immunity will endanger everyone is without validity.

Medical care is an individual question in a free country. Medical practice has a tendency to follow traditions long after they are useful. Vaccinations should be a question for each individual to answer. Only then will we be free to be healthy.

MORE ON IMMUNIZATIONS

Dear *Mothering,*

I have a 22-month-old son who will soon be due for his two-year-old checkup. I am advised by my pediatrician that at this checkup my son will have to take a new vaccine called *Hemophilus influenza* type b, or Hib vaccine, to prevent a common cause of bacterial meningitis in children from two to five years old. Any information from *Mothering* or help from other readers on this would be most appreciated. Thank you.

Dora Young
Houston, Texas

Editor's Note: Although this vaccine is "federally recommended," it is not required.

Hemophilus influenza *type b is the leading bacterial cause of meningitis, deep tissue infections, epiglottis, and diseases of the bones and joints. A child's risk of contracting one of these illnesses over the first five years of life is one in 200. Each year one out of 1,000 children are affected, 75 percent of them under the age of two. The current vaccine, however, is not effective in protecting them. It is administered to children at two years of age, although some pediatricians are recommending it at 18 months for children in playgroup settings. Thus, in the large cultural picture, this vaccine will theoretically prevent 25 percent of the H flu disease.*

The risks from the vaccine are, so far, reportedly low. Mild fevers and local reactions have been documented, with less than 1 percent of the recipients registering fevers greater than 101°. The only serious reaction documented has been an allergic response in one child who was then treated without complications.

According to effectiveness studies thus far, of those children who received the vaccine and were included in the study, 90 percent showed protective levels of antibodies.

Dear *Mothering,*

One of the major issues my husband and I have considered is immunizations. After reading all the *Mothering* articles on the subject and sending for the five outside sources advertised, we came to the decision not to have our daughter immunized.

I have strong feelings that it is in the best interest of my child and of future generations not to do this. However, it has never been an easy decision to live with. There are times when I suffer feelings of anxiety and paranoia at the thought of my child contracting one of the serious diseases, or viruses. What really *are* the risks of taking your child abroad to countries where these diseases are still present? What about the problem of letting her play with friends who have recently been given the live polio vaccine?

The hardest part is feeling very alone in this decision. None of our friends, so far, has made the same choice. Many were intimidated by the health-care workers, and now wish they'd been able to give it more thought. Our chiropractor is the only person we know who has given his children no immunizations, trusting in the healthy human body's ability to protect and heal itself.

I would like to appeal to anyone who shares our doubts

about vaccines to write to us. Let us know of your thoughts, feelings, information, and experiences. Does anyone know if homeopathic vaccines are in use anywhere today?

Sarah Watson
Suquamish, Washington

Dear *Mothering*,

I would like to share our family's experience with whooping cough. I am a naturopathic physician, and my wife is an RN. We have a daughter, age six, and a son, age four. Both have had better-than-average health, and neither has received any immunizations.

This fall our son developed a mild fever, which was followed by a cough that gradually worsened. About a week later, our daughter began to cough also. At first I thought that they had a viral bronchitis, and treated them with garlic extract, vitamins, and a dairyless wholesome diet. When the cough became more violent, with spasms occasionally ending in vomiting and sometimes the characteristic "whoop" for air between coughs, I had my son cultured and our suspicion of pertussis was confirmed.

Public school had just started the day before the lab report came back. We were faced with the likelihood of another four to six weeks of coughing (the typical length of the whooping stage). The public health officer would not allow our daughter to return to school until she had taken antibiotics for five days of a 14-day course to prevent her spreading it. Meanwhile, our daycare provider decided that she could not take the risk of caring for our unimmunized children. Except for a few friends, we felt alone and overwhelmed by the backlash of society's disapproval.

On the bright side, our children were doing fine. Between occasional coughing spasms they appeared and acted completely well. The worst coughing was at night. We agreed to and completed the full course of antibiotics so that our daughter could return to school. As antibiotics do not alter the course of pertussis but only reduce its communicability, we continued alternative therapies, adding the homeopathic *Drosera.* Over the next month, the coughs grew less frequent and severe. Our daughter missed only three days of school. Neither child had any complications or was hospitalized.

In retrospect, Diana and I do not regret our decision not to immunize; we affirm it. Pertussis is a serious disease with potentially serious complications, especially for infants. The pertussis bacteria is prevalent. Immunity from the vaccine lapses after several years, and adults can contract it and mistake it for a cold. The decision not to immunize carries with it a substantial risk of contracting the disease. We are relieved that our children are past it now and have natural immunity. For us, we feel we made the right decision.

The most difficult part of this experience was dealing with the social consequences of not immunizing. We had to put up with the hostility of local pediatricians, who viewed our initial decision as neglect; the disapproval of public health officials; our daughter's loss of her first days of school; and the social ostracism and eventual loss of our daycare provider. The lesson we learned is that we have to be willing to pay the price society extracts for us standing by our convictions.

Brent Mathieu, ND
Billings, Montana

MORE ON THE HIB VACCINE

Dear *Mothering,*

In answer to your letter in *Mothering,* no. 39 (Spring 1986), I'm also getting a lot of questions about the Hib vaccine. One reason why I think I'm receiving so many questions is because people are already suspicious about the old vaccines. Another reason stems from the behavior of physicians who have been taught to use a new remedy as quickly as possible before the side effects become known. Both parents and physicians already know that there is no such thing as a vaccine that has been proven safe and effective. Therefore, the concerns about this new vaccine, designed to protect children against *Hemophilus influenza* infections, meningitis included, are escalating.

I tell parents that when they are faced with the question of whether or not to give their child the Hib vaccine, they should read the prescribing information that the pharmaceutical company has prepared. You will learn that the maximum incidence of *Hemophilus influenza* meningitis occurs before the age of 18 months, whereas the vaccine is only supposed to be given after 24 months of age. You will learn that one shot does not confer enough protection; therefore, the doc-

tors are recommending booster shots. Yet, there is no deter-
mination thus far of the need
for booster shots or the frequency of the need for booster shots. You will also learn
that there are certain diseases
caused by the *Hemophilus influenza* germ—such as sinusitis, ear
infections, and a variety of others—that are not prevented by
vaccine. I therefore recommend against the Hib vaccine.

In addition, this vaccine
becomes especially suspect considering that, like every other
vaccine, no one has conducted a controlled study on it.
That is, no one has taken a
group of candidates, given half
of them the Hib vaccine, left the
other half alone (or given the
other half a placebo, like sugar-
water), and then compared
the outcomes (in terms of both
short-term and long-term effectiveness and damage) in the
two groups. In the absence of
this kind of study, the Hib vac-

cine remains an "unproven
remedy."

Robert S. Mendelsohn, MD
Evanston, Illinois

UNVACCINATED CHILDREN

Richard Moskowitz

Richard Moskowitz, MD, received his undergraduate degree from Harvard University and his medical degree from New York University before studying homeopathy with George Vithoulkas in Athens, Greece. He recently served as president of the National Center for Homeopathy in Washington, DC, and is the author of a book on homeopathy in pregnancy and birth to be published in 1993 by North Atlantic Press. A Contributing Editor to Mothering, *Dr. Moskowitz currently practices classical homeopathy in Watertown, Massachusetts. "Unvaccinated Children" first appeared in* Mothering, *no. 42 (Winter 1987).*

The refusal of significant numbers of parents to vaccinate their children has created a sizable group of people needing very much to be studied, and has raised a number of important public health issues. Foremost among them is the fear that a large reservoir of unvaccinated persons could contribute to epidemic outbreaks that might involve vaccinated individuals as well. Equally pressing are the immediate practical questions of how best to protect the unvaccinated persons from disease, how to prevent such outbreaks if possible, and how to treat them effectively if they do occur.

The long-term question which interests me the most is what the general health of this unvaccinated group will be like, and what we can deduce from this data concerning how vaccines really act.

I would like to begin by proposing that we use the terms *vaccinated* and *unvaccinated* instead of *immunized* and *unimmunized*, since the basis of the vaccination controversy is the belief of many parents that the vaccines do not produce a true *immunity*, but rather act in some other fashion—or, in my view, that they act *immunosuppressively*.

This may sound like a purely semantic distinction, but in fact it bears directly on the first question raised above. If the vaccines conferred a true immunity, as the natural illnesses do, then the unvaccinated people would pose a risk only to themselves. Children recovering from the measles or polio or whooping cough need never fear getting them again, no matter how often they are reexposed in the future. So, the reports of large-scale pertussis outbreaks in the United Kingdom since the vaccine was made optional seem to me a convincing argument against vaccinating *anybody*, even those who desire it, because if the vaccine produces authentic immunity, then this rebound phenomenon should not occur.

Furthermore, we should be skeptical about the "outbreaks" that are reported to have occurred. Pertussis, or whooping cough, is actually rather difficult to diagnose conclusively, as it requires special cultures or antibody tests that many laboratories cannot perform and that many doctors, in the presence of suggestive symptoms, rarely take the trouble to order. Conversely, there are other cases of pertussis with typical signs and symptoms but negative cultures and no detectable antibodies. In other words, whooping cough as a clinical *syndrome* need not be associated with the organism *Bordetella pertussis*, against which the vaccine is prepared, or indeed with any microorganism whatsoever.

Reservoirs of people unvaccinated against measles, mumps, or diphtheria, on the other hand, *should* result in periodic outbreaks of these diseases. But again, authentic immunity would ensure that *only* the unvaccinated would fall ill, which has never proved to be the case. All known outbreaks of these diseases in the postvaccine era have included large numbers of vaccinated people as well; and in many instances a large *majority* of the cases had previously been vaccinated, some of them quite recently.

The argument that parents should vaccinate their children to protect society as a whole from epidemics does not make sense. Such epidemics argue rather *against* vaccinating the ones who *were* vaccinated but still came down with the disease as soon as they were exposed to it. Likewise, if we accept partial or temporary immunity—conceding that the vaccines are not that effective, but that we have no other alternative to these rebound epidemics—then are we not simply throwing good lives after bad, rather like acknowledging that our patients are addicted to dangerous drugs yet fearing to withdraw such drugs or even withhold them from others, lest the original error be fully or frankly exposed?

Which brings us to the second question, namely, how to protect your unvaccinated child from an acute outbreak of one of these illnesses in the vicinity. The first priority is clearly to *know the illness*—its signs and symptoms, its natural history and vehicles of dissemination, its prevention and treatment.

Rather than reading this information from a pediatrics text and then passing it along to you, I suggest that you read up on these diseases. Even more importantly, meet with your local pediatrician or primary healthcare provider and plan a course of action. If you cannot immediately find someone whom you can work with or relate to, *keep looking*. Your local support system is too important to be left for the time when you need help in a hurry.

Taking responsibility for not vaccinating is no different from taking responsibility for a homebirth or any other form of alternative health care. It calls not for a substitute for conventional care, but rather a different *relationship* to the healing process and the healthcare system, based on personal choice and direct participation. We still need help when our children get sick, and we need to know that this help is available to us.

In the event of an outbreak, a great deal can be done to minimize the risk to those exposed and to treat those who actually fall ill—much of which does not involve chemical drugs or

vaccines of questionable safety and effectiveness. The homeopathic method, one such approach, uses minute doses of natural substances to stimulate and enhance the natural defense
mechanisms of the host. The homeopathic prevention and
treatment of specific acute diseases are discussed in detail in the
highly recommended book *Homeopathy in Epidemic Diseases* by
Dr. Dorothy Shepherd, a prominent English homeopath.[1]

The homeopathic approach to epidemic diseases in general
was first employed by Samuel Hahnemann in 1799, during an
extensive scarlet fever epidemic in the province of Saxony.[2] After
he had treated a dozen or so cases in the usual homeopathic fashion, giving small doses of remedies capable of *producing* similar
illnesses experimentally, Hahnemann realized that one remedy
helped to cure at least 75 percent of the cases, a second remedy covered another 15 percent or so, and the remaining 10
percent required a variety of different remedies corresponding
to the unique features of each case. The principal remedy,
which corresponded to the *genus epidemicus* (the main charac-
teristics of the outbreak as a whole), was then given out *prophylactically* to people exposed to the disease, and also to patients
in the early stages of illness—before the critical point, when other
remedies would sometimes be needed, was reached.

The results were quite dramatic. Those so treated either did
not get sick at all or suffered much milder illnesses, on the whole,
than their compatriots who were not treated or who received
the drugs and other heroic measures in standard practice at the
time. Hahnemann became justly famous for this exploit; and
since this time, his method has been used with equal or greater
success throughout the world in treating numerous outbreaks

of cholera, typhus, smallpox, yellow fever, influenza, and other acute diseases of a similar type. Why it has not been more widely influential in this country is a great mystery, and clearly has to do with the historic decline of homeopathy as a *thought form* until the advent of the alternative health and self-care movement of the past 10 years or so.

Pertussis

Whooping cough can be quite a nasty and prolonged illness, even in older children, in whom it is seldom fatal or dangerous. It can certainly threaten life in young infants under one year of age, because of the narrowness of the immature laryngeal opening and its particular vulnerability to obstruction from any inflammation or swelling. It is rarely serious in children older than six; and adults, for some reason, rarely contract the illness at all, even when they are exposed and have never had it before.

The incubation period varies from one to two weeks; and the illness often begins quite slowly, with some fever, typical upper respiratory symptoms, and a cough that gradually becomes more and more paroxysmal, until the characteristic spasms appear, often terminating in vomiting or tenacious sputum ejected with great violence. Such a cough may commonly persist for six weeks or even longer, suggesting an autoallergic as well as an infectious origin.

The nosode *Pertussin*, prepared from the sputum of patients with this disease, is the homeopathic remedy generally used for prophylaxis of exposed children (*Pertussin* 30c, one dose daily for two weeks after contact); and it can also be given in early stages of illness, at four-hour intervals. *Drosera* is the remedy most often used for the illness itself, although other remedies may also be needed. For children with a well-developed cough, *Drosera* 30c or *Pertussin* 30c may be given every four hours, or even more often if necessary. A physician should be consulted if the illness is severe.

Homeopathic remedies are available without prescription, but care should be exercised to obtain them from a manufacturer belonging to the American Association of Homeopathic Pharmacies. This way, you will know that they have been prepared in accordance with the standards of the United States Homeopathic Pharmacopoeia.

Diphtheria

Diphtheria is rarely seen today in developed countries, but small outbreaks have occurred in the southwestern United States (San Antonio in 1977). The illness is primarily a *poisoning* attributable to the toxin (a highly antigenic protein of high molecular weight) elaborated by the diphtheria bacillus. Diphtheria toxin is the source from which the standard vaccine is prepared (diphtheria "toxoid" is the toxin denatured by heat, alum-precipitated, and preserved with an organomercury compound), and is also the source of the homeopathic remedy, or nosode, *Diphtherinum*, which is commonly used for prophylaxis and for treatment of complicated cases.

Diphtheria begins as a "cold" or sore throat after a very brief incubation period of two or three days. The primary infection is usually in the throat or nasopharynx, and quickly becomes apparent with a grayish, ulcerating "pseudomembrane," foul breath, high fever, and marked swelling of the cervical lymph nodes (producing the classic "bull neck" in severe cases). Complications such as heart or kidney failure or esophageal obstruction may follow within a few days; and severe cases may be accompanied by difficulty in swallowing or talking, due to residual post-diphtheritic paralysis that may require further treatment. *Diphtherinum* 30c or 200c may be given in a daily dose for the first three days following exposure. A physician should be consulted and other remedies used if the illness develops.

Tetanus

Tetanus is essentially a *wound infection* complicated by inoculation of tetanus spores into the wound and germination of these under strict *anaerobic* conditions. The infection itself is relatively minor; like diphtheria (and its close relative botulism), tetanus is largely an *intoxication* produced by a highly antigenic protein, tetanus toxin, against which the standard vaccine is prepared by heat denaturation.

Tetanus does not occur epidemically, and cannot be passed from person to person, although conditions associated with wound infections (such as warfare) definitely favor it if the spores are present. The spore-forming organisms live in horse manure, and to a lesser extent in human manure (chiefly among people who keep horses); but the spores themselves are highly weather-resistant and can survive in the soil for decades. They will germinate only under strict anaerobic conditions—such as a deep, jagged puncture wound with enough tissue damage to get the infection started (the proverbial "rusty nail") or a simple wound infection (a severe burn or an infected umbilical cord stump in a newborn) that consumes all the available oxygen and thereby allows the spores to germinate underneath.

Careful attention to wound hygiene will effectively eliminate the possibility of tetanus in the vast majority of puncture wounds. Wounds should be carefully inspected, thoroughly cleaned, surgically debrided of dead tissue (under local anesthesia, if necessary), and not allowed to close until healing is well under way "from below." Two homeopathic remedies that may have a useful role at this stage are *Ledum* 30c, which should be given every two to four hours from the time of the puncture, and *Hypericum* 30c, which should be substituted if any signs of infection are present.

I have had no experience with *Tetanus*, the remedy prepared from the toxin itself; and tetanus toxoid is of no value unless the individual has previously been vaccinated, since a primary antibody response takes at least 14 days, and the incubation period of the disease can be considerably shorter than this (three to 14 days). *Hypericum* can reputedly treat as well as prevent tetanus, but I would recommend giving human antitoxin at the first sign of the disease, since it is far less effective later on.

If you do decide to vaccinate your children with tetanus toxoid alone, there is no need to vaccinate until the child is old enough to walk around and navigate on his or her own (18 to 24 months), at which time the vaccine is far less likely to cause complications.

Poliomyelitis

The poliovirus produces no illness at all in over 90 percent of those exposed to it; among others, it causes, at most, an ordinary flu syndrome with fever, weakness, gastrointestinal symptoms, aches, and pains. Even in epidemic conditions, poliomyelitis (the severe central nervous system complication) develops only in relatively few anatomically susceptible persons, most of whom eventually recover.

The typical symptoms of poliomyelitis include extreme sensitivity to touch, irritability, stiff neck, and fine tremors in the early or preparalytic stage, which may look rather like a viral meningitis. Not infrequently, the fever will return to normal for a few days just prior to the onset of these central nervous system symptoms, at which time it will rise again, producing the "dromedary," or double-hump, fever chart. Paralysis—due to inflammation of the anterior horn cells, or motor nuclei of the spinal cord—often appears suddenly and early in the course of the illness, as complete loss of voluntary movement in a single limb, or perhaps of the palate and throat muscles (in the dangerous brain-stem or bulbar type), producing disturbances of swallowing. Most of these cases will still recover, with residual paralysis or death often supervening much later, after the acute inflammation has subsided.

The homeopathic remedy *Lathyrus sativus* has been found to correspond most closely in its symptomatology to central nervous system polio, and has been used with great effectiveness both for prophylaxis of exposed individuals and for treatment in the early stages of the illness, before irreversible damage has occurred. According to Dr. Shepherd, a Dr. Taylor Smith of Johannesburg used *Lathyrus* 30c, one dose every 16 days, in 82 healthy people (aged six months to 20 years) living in a seriously infected area, 12 of whom were direct contacts. This regimen was continued for the duration of the outbreak, and not one of these people developed poliomyelitis.

Dr. Smith also used *Lathyrus* 30c in three doses, 30 minutes apart, for a second group of 34 children who were ill with fever, neck rigidity, and muscle tenderness of varying severity. All of these children recovered promptly and completely, without any sequelae.

Dr. Grimmer of Chicago, a well-known homeopath of the 1930s and 1940s, recommended *Lathyrus* 30c or 200c in a single dose repeated every three weeks for the duration of the epidemic, and stated most emphatically, from his own experience, that paralysis will *not* develop in those so treated. Other remedies may be required for the illness itself, at the first sign of which a physician should, of course, be consulted.

Measles

Wild-type measles is a strong, febrile illness lasting at least one or two weeks, with a long incubation period of 14 to 21 days; a characteristically smooth, confluent rash; "measly" or runny catarrh of eyes and nose; and a sizable risk of further developments, such as pneumonia, otitis media, or even laryngitis of the croupy or whooping cough type. The incidence of measles in susceptible contacts approaches 100 percent; and in populations not previously exposed to it, the fatality rate may be 20 percent or more. After generations of contact with European and North American cultures, it became a largely self-limited illness for these populations, one still memorable but producing complete recovery and a permanent or lifelong immunity in the vast majority of cases.

The prophylaxis and treatment of measles varies somewhat from outbreak to outbreak, the *genus epidemicus* corresponding most closely to *Pulsatilla* in Hahnemann's series, *Bryonia* in Dr.

Shepherd's experience, and probably other remedies in other times and places. In the United States, largely because of mass vaccination programs, acute measles is now predominantly a disease of adolescents and young adults, undoubtedly involving some genetic interaction with the vaccine virus; and it will probably call for still other remedies. *Pulsatilla* remains the remedy most often recommended for prophylaxis, although my own experience is still too limited to confirm or refute it.

Mumps

Mumps, or epidemic parotitis, resembles measles in its highly contagious nature and its predilection for the older age groups as a result of the vaccine program; but it is milder, as a rule. After an incubation period of three weeks, it begins with fever, runny nose, tenderness around the ears, and swelling of the parotid on one side, spreading to the other in a few days. About 25 percent of boys with mumps show swelling and inflammation of one or both testicles; in girls, the ovaries and breasts are occasionally affected. Residual scarring and atrophy of one testicle is sometimes seen in adolescent boys and young men.

The nosode *Parotidinum*, prepared from the saliva of an infected individual, may be used prophylactically, although *Pilocarpine* 6c is the remedy recommended by Shepherd for both prevention and treatment. I have had no personal experience using remedies with mumps.

Rubella

Rubella, or German measles, is the mildest of all the illnesses for which vaccines are presently required, and very often escapes

detection entirely. In the adolescent and young adult populations—those presently most likely to develop it—the illness
may be somewhat bothersome, with arthritic symptoms more
likely; the same symptoms are often encountered after vaccination
of these age groups. In children, there is no reason to treat rubella at all, in most cases. Pregnant women, especially those
exposed in the first trimester, may be given *Pulsatilla* 6c or 30c
every day for 14 days following exposure, or every four hours
for fever and acute symptoms. Rubella should be suspected in
the event of a mild fever; punctate rash; and swollen or tender
lymph nodes behind the ears and neck, and around the base
of the skull—an area seldom affected in other ailments.

People often ask if it is possible to "vaccinate" homeopathically, to use remedies for the same purpose that the vaccines
are normally given. This question addresses not short-term
prophylaxis in the event of an acute outbreak, which is discussed
above, but routine, long-term protection of the entire population against these diseases.

There is some evidence that remedies can be used in this way.
I know of several British veterinarians who use homeopathic rabies
nosode in lieu of injections to protect their dogs—with no serious side effects and, as yet, no rabies. But in order to do so, they
must give the remedy repeatedly throughout the life of the animal—an approach that would be much less suitable for humans.
This brings us back to the concept of trying to permanently eliminate susceptibility to specific diseases. Why attempt such an uneco-
nomical fantasy, as well as an unnecessary one, since the remedies work so splendidly well when illness is actually present or
threatening?

People also ask whether or not homeopathic treatment can be used in conjunction with vaccines. Homeopathic remedies may be given to mitigate the effect or severity of vaccines, just as they have been used with good effect in cases of vaccine-related illness. Certainly, when vaccines *are* given, I would recommend giving *Ledum* 30c—the basic first-aid remedy for puncture wounds—immediately afterward, in three doses 30 minutes apart; and following them with either the nosode prepared from the disease or vaccine itself or *Thuja* 30c, the general "antidote" to all vaccines, in three doses 12 hours apart.

Be aware of the possibility that a strong family history of vaccine reaction may greatly increase the risk of receiving that particular vaccine. Any child whose brother or sister or parent reacted strongly or violently to a vaccine should certainly be excused from receiving it, preferably by obtaining a medical exemption from a physician practicing in that state. Likewise, any child whose sibling or parent previously contracted poliomyelitis, or a severe or complicated case of measles or whooping cough or any of the other diseases listed, should not receive the vaccine prepared against that illness. Other grounds for medical exemption include preexisting epilepsy, central nervous system disorder, or any severe or disabling chronic disease where the risk of serious exacerbation from the vaccine outweighs the more imponderable long-term benefit.

This brings us to the final question of the long-term impact of mass vaccination programs on individual and community health. Since I have expressed my concerns on this score,[3] many people have asked if any research has been done to substantiate them. I can only appreciate the irony in the fact that the *compulsory* feature of these programs is precisely what makes it so conveniently impossible to study them—so much so that parents refusing to vaccinate their children deserve to be congratulated for making such research possible, and should, in fact, be recruited when it is ready to be carried out.

Equally noteworthy are the unprecedented breadth and scope of the research that will be required. Nothing less than the total health picture of vaccinated and unvaccinated children, followed over an entire generation, will suffice—a great collective enterprise that not only will be exciting and important in itself, but surely will yield invaluable new models for holistic medical research generally, models that will take us well beyond the outmoded focus on single "disease entities" in which we are still imprisoned today. So, regardless of whether or not you decide to vaccinate, I urge you all to think about a mechanism for how collaborative research of this kind can be conducted, and how each of us can play our part in it.

Notes

1. Dorothy Shepherd, MD, *Homeopathy in Epidemic Diseases* (Rustington, Essex [U.K.]: Health Sciences Press, 1967). Available from Homeopathic Educational Services, 2124 Kittredge St., Berkeley, CA 94704.
2. Samuel Hahnemann, MD (1755–1843), the discoverer of homeopathy.
3. Richard Moskowitz, "The Case against Immunizations," *Journal of the American Institute of Homeopathy 76* (7 March 1983). Abridged version published in *Mothering*, no. 31 (Spring 1984).

VACCINE UPDATE

Confusion surrounds the vaccination question, and the debate continues. Some illnesses that we routinely vaccinate against are virtually nonexistent in this country. Diphtheria is apparently absent from the United States, with no cases reported in 1986. Only three cases had been reported in the two years previous to that. Reported tetanus cases totaled 61 in 1986, and only two cases of paralytic poliomyelitis were reported in 1986.

Pertussis, however, despite near universal vaccination, was more prevalent in 1986 than in any year since 1970. The 1986 total number of pertussis cases was approximately 4,500, with nearly a third of them—1,300 cases—reported in a major outbreak in Kansas. (All 1986 statistics cited above are from the provisional data compiled by the Centers for Disease Control and reported in *Vaccine Bulletin*, February 1987, pp. 11–12.)

This outbreak of pertussis in Kansas occurred in a highly immunized population: "Some 90 percent of the pertussis patients whose immunization status was known, appear to have been adequately immunized." (*Vaccine Bulletin*, February 1987, p. 11) The outbreak affected all age groups—from 0 to 79 years—with most cases concentrated in those under 20 years of age. More cases than would usually be expected occurred in the five to nine age group, and less than would be expected occurred among infants.

Vaccine complications continue to receive national press coverage. Some attention has been given to the development of a different type of vaccination for pertussis, one that is associated with fewer vaccine-related complications. The pertussis vaccine currently in use in this country is a *whole-cell* vaccine, which contains dead pertussis toxin—that remains biologically active after the bacteria that secrete it have been killed—as well as endotoxin, a protein secreted by a virus or bacteria that can, in large enough quantities, affect the brain or produce shock. Developed several years ago in Japan, the *acellular* pertussis vaccine has all of the bacteria and most of the tox-

ins removed or rendered harmless, and is considered more pure and specific. Although the acellular vaccine must undergo testing in this country and physicians will not have legal access to it for two to three years, some physicians who are concerned about side effects from the whole-cell preparation are using test batches of the new vaccine for their own children or are traveling to Japan or Hong Kong to have their children vaccinated. (*The Santa Fe New Mexican*, 5 April 1987)

Two preliminary studies of the acellular vaccine in the United States show promising results. Vanderbilt University School of Medicine and the UCLA School of Medicine have thus far conducted studies on 80 children from 18 to 24 months and from four to six years of age. Both age groups showed antibody production comparable to the old vaccine, but far fewer adverse reactions in terms of fever, fretfulness, abnormal gait, and redness, tenderness, and swelling at the vaccination site. (*Healthfacts*, no. 90, November 1986)

Among the non-Communist countries, only the United States, Australia, and Iceland have mandatory pertussis vaccination programs. And yet, the pertussis inoculation is the most toxic of all protective vaccines routinely given to children in their first five years of life. Each year, this vaccine is linked to the deaths of at least 44, and possibly as many as 900, otherwise healthy children. It also causes more lasting brain damage than whooping cough would if children were not immunized. Most of the whooping cough in America now occurs in vaccinated children or in those too young to be immunized. (*The Santa Fe New Mexican*, 5 April 1987)

Both Sweden and Japan experienced an increase in cases of whooping cough after discontinuing mass whole-cell vaccination programs. Japan, now using the acellular vaccine and waiting until two years of age to begin vaccination has witnessed a dramatic decline in both minor and severe reactions to the vaccine and in cases of whooping cough in general. (*The People's Medical Journal*, December 1986)

Many questions remain to be answered regarding the relationship between vaccinations and the decline of an illness in the general population over time; the effect of vaccinations on the immune system; and the safety of administering particular vaccines in a country in which diseases from the conditions vaccinated against are on the decline and in which large numbers of vaccinated people still contract the disease.

Ellen Kleiner
Good News

MENINGITIS VACCINE UPDATE

In *Mothering*, no. 39 (Spring 1986), we printed a letter from a reader inquiring about the Hib vaccine, licensed in the United States in April 1985 to protect against the leading bacterial cause of meningitis. Since then, more research has shed light on the problem and on the vaccine. Two recent studies have concluded that *Hemophilus influenza* type b does not seem to spread from child to child as readily as doctors suspected. (*New England Journal of Medicine*) Earlier studies indicated that the infant brothers or sisters of a child with meningitis are up to 400 times more likely to contract this illness; however, one of the more recent studies showed that only one child out of 587 who had regular contact with an infected toddler went on to develop the illness.

Vaccine failure is also being investigated. Work is under way to determine why it is that some children who receive the preparation go on to develop meningitis. (*New England Journal of Medicine 315*, 18 December 1986)

All we can conclude at this point is that contact with meningitis is less "risky" than was formerly believed; that the other causes of meningitis (such as pneumococcus, meningococcus, some viruses, and other agents) are not inoculated against in the current vaccine; that the Hib vaccine is not effective in the under-two age group, in which 75 percent of all meningitis cases occur; and that the current vaccine will not protect all children who receive it.

Ellen Kleiner
Good News

VACCINE REFORM IN ALASKA

Vaccination reform legislation is under way in Alaska. Representative Mike Navarre presented HB 277, an act relating to the inoculation of minors to the Alaska State House on 17 April 1987. The bill has been referred to the Health, Education, and Social Services Committee and will be reviewed when the House of Representatives reconvenes in January 1988.

This bill has four main components. *Parental Choice:* To allow philosophical objection (parental discretion) on administration of vaccinations without threat of exclusion from a school, preschool, or daycare center. *Parent Immunization Information:* To mandate that each parent receive extensive written information on the risks as well as the benefits of each vaccine before vaccination and with vaccine information provided by the Public Health Department at birth. *Adverse Reaction Reports:* To mandate that all healthcare providers report to the Public Health Department all occurrences of serious adverse reactions resulting from inoculations, and that long-term follow-up investigations be included. *Immunization Records:* To ensure that the vaccine manufacturer and lot number be kept on file for at least three years, and that reactions be recorded in a minor's permanent medical record so that no further doses of questionable vaccine are administered to that minor, even if location of administration varies.

Alaska—Dissatisfied Parents Together (AK-DPT) is requesting that all concerned Alaskan parents contact their representatives and ask them to support HB 277. Address letters to Representative _____, AK State Legislature, Pouch V (MS 3100), Juneau, AK 99811. Public support is the key to passage of this much needed legislation.

Readers interested in learning more about these proceedings may contact: Shannon Kohler, President, AK-DPT, Box 1746, Soldotna, AK 99669.

Ellen Kleiner
Good News

MENINGITIS VACCINE: CONTROVERSIAL FINDINGS

In last summer's issue of *Mothering* (Summer 1987), we printed an update on the vaccine that was approved by the Federal Drug Administration (FDA) in April 1985 to protect against *Hemophilus influenza* type b (Hib), the leading bacterial cause of meningitis. The Centers for Disease Control (CDC) recommended essentially universal vaccination for children at 24 months of age. This past October, the Infectious Disease Committee of the American Academy of Pediatrics (AAP) approved alternative guidelines: under certain circumstances, physicians may choose not to use this vaccine.

The "certain circumstances" are based on recent studies of the vaccine's efficacy and safety in different parts of the country. Five retrospective studies presented at an FDA workshop this past April showed a "surprising number of meningitis cases" among children who had received the vaccine. And Dan Granoff, a pediatrician at Washington University's Children's Hospital in St. Louis, has commented on the vaccine's "unprecedented regionality." In Minnesota, for example, vaccinated children were *more* likely than nonvaccinated children to become infected with Hib; those who became infected were 86 percent more likely than controls to have been vaccinated. (*Science News 132*, 24 October 1987)

Minnesota State epidemiologist Michael Osterholm claims that, rather than protecting children from meningitis, the Hib vaccine increases the risk of illness. He reported that a Minnesota study of children who had received the vaccine since its introduction in 1985 showed they faced a fivefold increase in the risk of infection by the Hib bacteria. ("Meningitis Risk Seen from Use of Vaccine," *St. Paul Pioneer Press Dispatch*, 21 April 1987) According to Granoff, these findings suggest that the vaccine might best be discontinued in this state.

Previous to this, researchers had never seen such regional variation in a vaccine's effectiveness. The original vaccine trials were conducted in Finland, where a 90 percent effectiveness rate was reported. Follow-up effectiveness trials in the United States have ranged from 89 percent in some states to the negative correlation found in Minnesota. Some physicians are now questioning the value of transferring data derived from countries with a homogeneous population to the more genetically diverse United States.

Also questionable is a particular person's susceptibility to the infection, regardless of his or her vaccination status. Studies among unvaccinated populations show that certain ethnic groups—blacks, American Indians, and Eskimos—are more susceptible to Hib infection than Caucasians. Other studies reveal that some vaccinated individuals seem completely incapable of mounting immune responses against Hib.

Consequently, new approaches to meningitis protection are under way. One development is a *conjugate vaccine* which, unlike the original preparation that is made from a polysaccharide fragment of the virus, will link this fragment to "immune system stimulants capable of amplifying antibody production." Researchers are hoping that conjugate vaccines will prove effective in children as young as six months of age. However, conjugate vaccines also have potential problems. One is that they have been pretested in Finland and not in this country. Another is that they have a "window of increased susceptibility" to Hib infection during the first seven days after inoculation. Granoff and others claim this is due to the vaccine's action of temporarily "binding up the body's naturally occurring Hib antibodies."

A second new development is *passive vaccination*. The passive vaccine, designed to provide rapid protection against infection, involves the direct injection of Hib-specific immune proteins (immune globulins) taken from the plasma of previously inoculated adults. The disadvantages are: it is expensive; protection is only temporary, requiring repeated doses; and it involves a human blood product and thus carries a small risk of hepatitis or AIDS contamination. (*Science News 132*, 24 October 1987)

As this issue goes to press, new guidelines are being formulated. On February 17, the AAP released a statement recommending that children receive the new conjugate vaccine (PRP-D) at 18 months of age in lieu of the "first-generation" polysaccharide (PRP) vaccine at 24 months. The new vaccine, licensed by the FDA this past December, is expected to be safer and more immunologic, and to offer protection to an additional 5 percent of children. The vaccine is not licensed for use in children under 18 months, an age group that encompasses 70 percent of all meningitis cases. (AAP News Release, 17 February 1988)

Ellen Kleiner
Good News

Excerpted from:

MOTHERING INTERVIEWS— RICHARD MOSKOWITZ

Mothering: *Are there any vaccinations that you like? Do you have any differences of opinion about the polio, tetanus, or pertussis vaccines?*

Moskowitz: I have mostly questions. My basic feeling about vaccinations revolves around questions more than answers; and those questions are so insistent and so pressing that I feel they must be answered. Until they are, I cannot subscribe to the practice of compulsory vaccinations. Routine "immunization" across the board, regardless of the individual's need or sensitivity, is producing high amounts of chronic disease in our population.

My sense is that vaccinating transforms the propensity to get acute diseases into the propensity to get chronic diseases. On the whole, I would much rather take my chances with the acute diseases. With chronic diseases, suffering is amortized over time; you pay for it over the course of your life.

We have to ask how vaccines affect the total health of individuals over a period of 15 or 20 years. However, we do not yet have the conceptual tools to do this, because we do not agree on what the total health of an individual is.

Infectious diseases come and go; they are part of the biosphere. To think that we can simply eliminate them through some kind of technical engineering is incredibly reckless. I think we are stepping into the genetic engineering department here, and that is a very dangerous thing to do. Vaccines are engineering changes in the genetic material that we really do not understand. I would prefer to accept the reality of sickness—to accept the fact that we do fall ill and that healing is possible.

Mothering: *Are unvaccinated people traveling in other countries more susceptible to illness?*

Moskowitz: This is currently up for grabs. I would hate to come down with yellow fever, for example. It is a very nasty sickness. But on the other hand, at this point in my life, I would be much more inclined to trust my own healing power, and whatever healers I would hope to find, than to trust the vaccine to protect me against yellow fever. I do not trust it anymore. I have come too far. As much as I would like to be able to trust it, I see the potential cost, and in some cases I have seen the actual cost. I am having to reexamine even vaccinations like tetanus toxoid. I just have these questions, and they will not go away.

Peggy O'Mara

MORE ON VACCINATIONS

Dear *Mothering,*

The most treasured part of my *Mothering* magazines are the letters. Living as I do, amidst another culture in an isolated area of Alaska, I regard the letters as my main chance to communicate with other like-minded mothers. In that spirit, I'd like to share my experience with vaccinations.

When our firstborn (now nearly four) received his first series of vaccinations at two months, my husband and I were only vaguely aware of the possible consequences of the DPT and were surprised at our son's reaction. For at least 12 hours he cried (except when nursing or sleep-ing), held his body rigid, and gave us no visual recognition. Before the next shot was due, we read a lot about vaccinations and were shocked that the doctor (who was filling in for our regular pediatrician) had given no explanation of known reactions and never asked us about our family history.

We discussed our concerns with our regular doctor. She said she would give our son the DT (DPT minus the pertussis) if we insisted, but she felt there was no medical reason for this and made a reference to people who worried a lot.

Finally, given what we knew about the possible benefits and

risks, and given our remote location—a plane trip away from a doctor or hospital, weather permitting—and the fact that several cases of pertussis had been diagnosed in our region, we decided to get our son vaccinated with DPT again. He is now "up to date" with his shots, and aside from mild fever, he has not had another observable reaction.

Still, we worried about what might happen when he received the final booster before starting school. We found a new doctor after our second son was born eight months ago. Before I consented to DPT shots for him, I wanted to find out if this doctor thought our older son's reaction was unusual. He thought the reaction was "neurological" and said he would *not* have taken a chance and given the pertussis to our child again. This information is now part of my son's medical record, and he will never have another pertussis shot.

For the reasons noted above, and because neither we nor our doctor were convinced that siblings necessarily react the same way, we had our younger son immunized with the full DPT series. He's had three inoculations, with no observable reaction.

The lesson for us and maybe for others is this: making decisions is much harder than remaining ignorant. Our decision to immunize was an informed one, and we were glad we were able to consider so many factors. Most importantly, we learned to trust our own instincts. Although our oldest son had none of the classic pertussis reactions, such as high-pitched screaming or convulsions, we felt his reactions weren't "normal" either. To think we risked his health three times before finding a doctor who agreed with us is frightening.

Alida Ciampa
Kiana, Alaska

Dear *Mothering*,

Over the years I have followed with great interest your articles on vaccines. After my firstborn's many bad reactions, I am inclined not to vaccinate my second child. But I am very concerned about the risks. Having conducted a lot of research on the vaccines and diseases, I am still looking for support for my decisions. Are there other parents who would be willing to share their grown children's health histories after choosing *not* to vaccinate?

Jane Stephens
La Conner, Washington

CHILDHOOD VACCINE EXEMPTIONS

Allowable exemptions to mandatory inoculations come in three forms: medical, religious, and philosophical. Medical exemptions, accepted in all 50 states, require a written statement from a licensed physician indicating that the particular vaccination is contraindicated due to a previous adverse reaction, a family history of reactions, a history of convulsions, neurological disorders, severe allergies, prematurity, or recent illness. Licensed naturopathic physicians in Washington State are now allowed to furnish medical exemptions, as are chiropractors in some states.

Religious exemptions are accepted in all states except West Virginia and Mississippi. Philosophical exemptions, based on a parent's personal beliefs, are permitted in 22 states. This option requires a written statement from the parent indicating that he or she has "a moral conviction opposed to vaccination." (Richard Leviton, "Who Calls the Shots?" *East West Journal,* November 1988)

As more parents claim religious exemptions for their children—particularly in states that do not allow philosophical exemptions—the legal system is having to acknowledge a wider range of beliefs. In a recent New York Federal Court lawsuit

(*Levy, et al. v. Northport–East North-port Union Free School District, et al.*), US District Court Judge Leonard Wexler ruled that parents can legally claim an exemption from inoculation based on their own "personal religious beliefs" and need not be members of any particular religious group. The earlier statute, requiring membership in a recognized religious organization, was declared unconstitutional—in violation of the First Amendment of the Constitution.

This case has expanded an individual's rights to refuse vaccination in New York. Now, says attorney James Filenbaum, who filed the suit, the courts will have to determine what constitutes "personal religious beliefs." (*Health Science,* November/ December 1988, p. 4)

For information on this ruling, contact attorney James Filenbaum, 300 N. Main Street, Suite 108, Spring Valley, NY 10977; 914-425-8804.

Ellen Kleiner
Good News

MORE ON VACCINATIONS, PERTUSSIS, AND TETANUS

Dear *Mothering*,

In response to Jane Stephens (Winter 1989), I chose not to have my son immunized, and his health is excellent. He is 11 years old, has never had an ear infection, is rarely sick at all, and is robust and thriving. His health is much better than his cousins' or than mine was as a child.

When he was a baby in 1978, I studied the pros and cons of immunization and concluded that my decision could not be based on intellectual thought alone. The literature for immunization is fear-based and does not admit to doubts of efficacy or the possibility of adverse side effects. The literature against immunization is also fear-based, sometimes hysterical. The challenge has been to find the middle way.

After much exploration, I decided to mother my child in ways that bolstered his health and strengthened his immune system naturally, reducing his risk of contracting illness as well as reducing the severity of illness if he were to get, say, whooping cough. Much harder for me to live with would be the consequences of vaccine damage, incurred by voluntarily submitting to an intrusive and questionable procedure. Iatrogenic problems, because they are rooted in ignorance, present a greater threat to me than the conditions they attempt to avoid.

I massage my son and my new four-month-old baby regularly, using Swedish, pressure point, and Reiki styles. We work with breath, visualization, emotional clearing, and Bach flower remedies. We all receive regular chiropractic care. Research has shown that regular massage doubles the levels of antibodies in the immune system. Metabolizing stress goes a long way toward creating and maintaining health. We are aware of the preconditions of illness, and we respond to them by making an effort to regain balance.

Two years ago, against my wishes, my ex-husband had our son, then nine, partially immunized. He had a topical reaction of redness, soreness, and heat at the site of the injection and ran a low fever. Subsequently, he showed symptoms of allergies for the first time ever.

I object deeply to the way vaccines are created—inflicting pain, disease, and degradation on animals. That energy is also present in the vaccines. The possible benefits of vaccination are outweighed by the brutality engendered in their manufacture.

I have never had any problems enrolling my son in preschool or public elementary school because of his not being immunized. I have, on numerous occasions, been severely criticized—by pediatricians and even close friends threatened by the idea that their children's health is not protected unless everyone is immunized. I am sure there are better ways to build immunity to dangerous diseases. Homeopathy is not a legally recognized branch of medicine in Texas, so our family turns to a holistic chiropractor for preventive health maintenance.

The wisdom of introducing

potent toxins directly into the bloodstream, where they have easy access to major organs, is questionable. The efficacy of vaccines, using World Health Organization statistics that are controlled for public health measures such as clean water, adequate food, and sewage control, is also questionable. The pedantic rigidity of the medical establishment is well documented, as is the unaccountability of drug manufacturers and individual doctors administering vaccines.

We parents and our children have to live with the consequences of their actions and our own. If we follow our hearts, we can do that, and we can learn from our mistakes. It could be that vaccination is a good alternative to the extensive lifestyle changes demanded by good preventive health habits and stress reduction.

Nancy Klein
Houston, Texas

Dear *Mothering*,

As a concerned parent, I feel the need to impress upon your readers the grave importance of the DPT series of immunizations. I had to deal with the consequences of my son's inability to tolerate the full DPT series when he contracted whooping cough at age 11 months. After three and a half weeks and many doctors, my son's respiratory system had been damaged. He was treated with erythromycin (after he was finally diagnosed), but erythromycin does nothing to the endotoxin produced by the pertussis bacteria, so we spent many sleepless months doing 24-hour respiratory therapy to ensure that our son would live. On several occasions, my son's inability to breathe caused "blue spells" while we could only wait helplessly for the paroxysms to subside. He now has asthma as a direct result of this disease.

Marcie Schonborn
Dallas, Texas

Dear *Mothering,*

I want to share our experience with whooping cough. I have two daughters, ages three years and five months. We live in a small isolated community of 1,500. Many people here came down with an endless coughing illness; some of them were immunized against pertussis, some were not. None was diagnosed as having pertussis. We found our local health professionals reluctant to test for whooping cough. I insisted, as my children are not immunized. Although I had been immunized as a child, my test was positive.

Even as more people came down with the coughing illness, no tests were done. Because they had been vaccinated against whooping cough, testing requests were refused. One friend who was eight months pregnant went in for a culture; when the doctor determined that she had been immunized, he refused to do the test. She has whooping cough and is due in three weeks.

Among all of our local cases, only a few had the "whoop" sound. We each had our own variation of the cough—all were bad. Some recovered in three weeks, whereas others are still coughing five months later.

My family took no antibiotics. We tried a homeopathic remedy without success. Our best bet seemed to be a good attitude (difficult when surrounded by fear and misinformation) coupled with months of garlic (crushed in a teaspoon with honey), echinacea tinctures, vitamin C, and multivitamins.

Whooping cough taught us temperance and patience. The illness is very long and not much fun to listen to or stay up all night with, but it was not life threatening for anyone in our community. It's an illness to be avoided, but I'm glad we went through it.

If the disease is detected early enough, a young child can pass through the illness safely. Whooping cough in a healthy person doesn't get that bad. Stress plays an important role. None of us turned blue, not even my infant who has a heart murmur.

A Loving Reader

Dear *Mothering*,

In all my reading about vaccinations, I have not come across much about tetanus shots. Assuming that vaccinations do work, this is the one shot I would consider for my 14-month-old son, since *Clostridium tetani* are so prevalent in animal feces and soil. Does anyone have references for or personal experiences with the disease and the effectiveness of its treatment or prevention by vaccinations? I would also be interested in personal accounts of successful treatment of the other diseases supposedly preventable by vaccinations.

Gabrielle Duebendorfer
Arcata, California

IMMUNIZATION:
THE REALITY BEHIND THE MYTH

Immunization: The Reality behind
  the Myth
Walene James
Bergin & Garvey Publishers
670 Amherst Road
South Hadley, MA 01075
1988, $10.95 paperback
  220 pages

There is much to like about this book and its author, and much to be grateful for. Ms. James is clearly knowledgeable, speaks from her heart, and makes her case against the philosophy, the practice, and the politics of vaccination in a most thorough, instructive, and sometimes eloquent fashion, incorporating a wealth of ideas from many different sources.

She touches all the bases: the scientific questions of efficacy, safety, and the nature of immunity in a broader context; the larger philosophical questions arising from the germ theory of disease (including the views of some of its original critics, now known mostly to historians of science); the contemporary political questions, originating in her own personal fight to exempt her two-year-old grandson from Virginia's compulsory vaccination requirements; and even her vision of a simpler and safer philosophy of healing.

The personal account was

especially moving and useful, because the child's parents didn't have the money to hire a fancy lawyer and were too principled and feisty to become nominal Christian Scientists and get "swept under the rug"; they squawked and hollered, contacted health workers, members of Congress, and lobbyists, and eventually *got it done.* That's what it takes, folks, and that's what it's going to take. People out there who don't want to vaccinate their kids, for whatever reason, will find much to learn in this book.

On the other hand, it probably will not change the minds of many who prefer to vaccinate or simply aren't sure. Make no mistake: the book is a *polemic,* an impassioned argument for a certain point of view, untroubled by doubt or even the slightest hint of skepticism about its conclusions. Nor does the author always bother to cite those whose ideas she paraphrases and digests and then regurgitates as if they were her own. Not an elegant piece of scholarly or scientific investigation, but the author's gutsy scrambling for her own personal truth— a truth that many others have chosen, are choosing, and will continue to choose to live by.

Richard Moskowitz, MD

VACCINE QUESTIONS

Dear *Mothering,*

After weeks of researching vaccinations, I've decided not to vaccinate my three-month-old daughter. I'm still undecided, however, about the polio vaccine. What concerns me is the risk of contagion from the vaccine itself. Most children in this country are being vaccinated with the live virus, which is excreted through their bowels for four to six weeks after the vaccine is given.

If an unvaccinated child is around a vaccinated child during these four to six weeks, what is the risk of contagion? Can the adult who changes the diapers carry the virus (from the vaccine)? What about all those dirty diapers? In cotton diapers, does the virus get killed in the wash, or does it go into the sewage system? In single-use diapers, how long does the virus live in the landfills? Are we in danger of it multiplying or seeping into the groundwater? Is this potential grounds for another epidemic, or will we stop administering this vaccine soon (as we did with the smallpox vaccine)?

I realize it would be mostly speculation, but I'm looking for facts, not paranoia. Does anyone know the scoop?

Nathalie Kelly
San Francisco, California

Dear Nathalie,

While I really do *not* have "the scoop," I will make a crude attempt to answer your excellent and thoughtful questions.

There is a risk of unvaccinated children acquiring live polio virus from the vaccinated ones, but it is difficult to quantify. At the very least, it's the perfect rejoinder to those who fear that their vaccinated children are at risk from the unvaccinated ones. There have been a few reported cases of polio in adults, mostly parents of vaccinated children, some severe. Furthermore, the religious fervor for vaccination is such that very little work is being done to assess the risk.

Second, you are quite right that people who change the diapers of vaccinated youngsters should wash their hands, and that the virus undoubtedly does find its way into the sewage (as it did in the celebrated epidemics of the 1950s). Also, the virus might persist in landfills and eventually find its way into the water supply. An epidemic of the vaccine virus (or some vaccine-wild type of hybrid) is also very possible.

Several people have asked me whether the risk of acquiring the virus from vaccinated children constitutes a reason for going ahead and vaccinating. That argument wholly fails to persuade me. The chance of getting the virus from your playmate is doubtless real, but the chance of getting it if you are vaccinated is a certainty!

Richard Moskowitz, MD
Contributing Editor
Jamaica Plain,
Massachusetts

Editor's Note: The American Academy of Pediatrics, in its Report of the Committee on Infectious Diseases (1988), states that "the OPV *[oral live polio vaccine] remains in the throat for one to two weeks and in the feces for several weeks, with a maximum excretion time of 60 days. Patients are potentially contagious as long as fecal excretion persists." According to the New Mexico State Department of Epidemiology, the virus is attenuated and potentially contagious only for immunosuppressed individuals.*

Dear *Mothering*,

This past year has seen the careful orchestration of the media by public health officials regarding measles "outbreaks" in order to enable them to obtain legislative mandates on second measles vaccination doses ("boosters") not only for our children but for adults as well, if we are 32 years old or younger. It is my understanding that 10 states have passed postsecondary student vaccination laws for mumps, measles, and rubella. What that amounts to is forced adult vaccination. I heard of no cases of college students opposing the vaccine—partly due to ignorance of the issue, and partly

because none of them was willing to give up credit for a class or forfeit a degree.

Public health officials and our legislators were able to push these bills through because there was no substantial public outcry or opposition. I urge *Mothering* supporters to write letters of opposition to the media so that the general public, politicians, and judges can see that there *is* opposition to the vaccination policy.

Bonnie Plumeri Franz
Ogdensburg, New York

Dear *Mothering*,

I would like to hear from other parents who decided against routine infant vaccination and then did some world travel with their children. What are the physiological implications of later vaccination against diseases that currently exist in other countries?

Dara Wishingrad
Montpelier, Vermont

VACCINATION QUESTIONS

Dear *Mothering*,

Long before I became pregnant with my son, I decided not to vaccinate. But after he was born, and after further thought and research, I decided to go ahead with the polio and tetanus vaccines. After his first polio shot at four months, Edward developed a diaper rash that persisted for two full months. He had never had a rash before. He has been fully breastfed, I use cloth diapers, and there has been no change in my diet. No prescribed, over-the-counter, or homeopathic cream has helped.

Now, after his second polio shot and first shot of tetanus,

Edward has developed hives. His pediatrician says that this is probably a reaction to the vaccines and that the diaper rash could be as well. He says that these are not reasons to discontinue the shots. But I'm not so sure. What if his next reaction is worse? Much worse?

I would appreciate hearing from anyone who has gone through a similar experience. What did you decide?

Alida Cynric
Madison, Wyoming

Dear *Mothering*,

After a great deal of agonizing and criticism from others, we have decided not to vaccinate our daughter Chloe. I feel good about this decision and have taken a lot of time to research it. I am worried, however, that she won't be able to contract the normal childhood diseases to develop her own natural immunities. How dangerous would it be if she got these diseases later in adolescence or adulthood? Are the consequences more serious? I'd be interested in hearing from anyone with answers to these questions or support for not vaccinating.

Gretchen Annie Wotzold
Tetonia, Idaho

TRAVELING WITHOUT VACCINES

Dear *Mothering,*

I would like to share my experience in traveling abroad with my nonvaccinated children. I have been living in Japan (where vaccination is suggested but not mandatory) for the past six years, and my two sons were born on Okinawa and in the Tokyo area. While traveling to and from the United States, I have never been questioned about the lack of vaccine records in my sons' passports. Because some diseases are more prevalent in countries other than the United States (such as cholera in Thailand and malaria in parts of Africa), I prefer to be careful with my family's overall health rather than accept the risks and questionable effectiveness of vaccines against these diseases. While in Kuala Lumpur and Bangkok, we drank only bottled water and ate at reputable restaurants. If necessary, I would accept the risks of disease over the risks of vaccination, or I would choose not to travel to certain disease-prone areas.

It is my understanding that under the WHO (World Health Organization) code, vaccines are not required upon entering countries that have disease-infested areas; however, a traveler may be quarantined for two weeks upon return to his or her country of origin. The quarantine may be as simple as returning home and reporting to a health official any symptoms found within the two-week period. This procedure may hold true for vaccinated as well as nonvaccinated individuals.

Jennifer Anne Schmidt
Kokubunji-shi, Japan

VACCINE UPDATES:
DPT, MEASLES, CHICKEN POX

Recent developments in vaccine research provide new food for thought. Data from the Centers for Disease Control (CDC) reaffirm that children receiving the DPT shot are at increased risk of having seizure. The analysts note that seizures may be either febrile (fever induced) or nonfebrile, and that children most at risk are those who have a first-degree relative with a history of convulsions. According to CDC estimates, if family history alone were used to disqualify children from the inoculation, 5 to 7 percent of youngsters in this country would not receive the DPT. (*The Journal of Pediatrics,* October 1989)

As these findings were going to press, a group of multidisciplinary scientists was convening for a three-day international symposium on pertussis—the "P" in DPT. Participants at the 28 September 1989 Workshop on the Neurological Complications of Pertussis and the Pertussis Vaccine concluded that the current whole-cell pertussis vaccine can cause a wide spectrum of permanent brain damage, ranging from learning disabilities to severe retardation to seizure disorders. According to workshop coordinator John Menkes, MD, a University of California at Los Angeles professor of pediatrics and neurology, the neurological complications are in part prompted by the interaction of pertussis toxin and the endotoxin present in B. pertussis bacteria. The scientists also concluded that whereas the vaccine may accelerate symptoms in children with an underlying neurologic disorder, *it can also produce symptoms in children with no preexisting abnormality.* Workshop attendants agreed on the importance of replacing the whole-cell vaccine with either a less toxic acellular vaccine or a genetically engineered preparation. (*Vaccine News 5*, no. 1, Spring 1990, pp. 1,9) A summary of key findings is available for $2.00 from The National Vaccine Information Center, Dissatisfied Parents Together (DPT), 204-F Mill St., Vienna, VA 22180; 703-983-DPT3.

Four months later, in a federal review of the pertussis vaccine, an Institute of Medicine panel of medical and public health experts maintained that although the vaccine can worsen preexisting problems and bring to light previously unknown problems, there is "no scientific proof that the vaccine causes severe neurological damage or death." Dissenting parents, lawyers, and others argued that public health officials, in their zealous promotion of mass inoculation to wipe out contagious diseases, are deliberately understating the severe side effects of the DPT vaccine. Jeffrey Schwartz—a Washington lawyer whose daughter's 1984 death was attributed to a vaccine-related seizure—pointed out that more than 1,000 reported cases of severe pertussis vaccine reactions are being brushed off by the medical community as "unscientific" and "anecdotal," and that the government, by withholding information about the danger of the vaccine, has been engaged in "a conspiracy of silence and denial." (*The Santa Fe New Mexican,* 11 January 1990, p. A–2)

On the measles front, in response to the nearly 400 percent increase in measles cases between 1988 and 1989, the American Academy of Pediatrics and the CDC are recommending revaccination of all individuals born after 1957. The reasoning is that "virtually everyone born before then was exposed to the highly contagious disease and is now immune to it," and the single shot most children have received since then "has not eradicated the disease." The two-dose recommendation was prompted by a desire to protect the 2 to 10 percent of children who have failed to respond to the first dose. Recommendations for newborns include a first dose of the vaccine at 15 months and a second dose before entering junior high school. Although

physicians say that measles is not serious in most cases, they note that it can "lead to life-threatening complications, including pneumonia and brain damage." (*The New York Times,* 30 July 1989, p. A–20)

The National Vaccine Information Center has raised several questions about the new measles protocol. First, considering the number of measles outbreaks in already vaccinated high school and college populations, could mass vaccinations have caused the measles virus to become more vaccine resistant? (And if so, could the new mass vaccination program create strains of even greater resistance?) Second, can revaccination be considered an effective option when no national study has been conducted to evaluate whether or not this two-dose option will provide lifelong immunity? And third, can revaccination be considered safe when no study has assessed whether or not the second dose of vaccine will result in adverse reactions? (*Vaccine News*, p. 9)

Another rash of measles concerns appears in Dr. Lisa Lovett's booklet *Immunity: Why Not Keep It?* Lovett presents documentation showing that since the introduction of the measles vaccine, death due to measles has not decreased, the incidence of pneumonia and demonstrable liver abnormalities has increased (from 3 to 20 percent), and children who die from measles are usually malnourished. She also highlights a 1983 study showing that half of all people with measles in the United States had been vaccinated against the disease. For a copy of this 74-page booklet, write to Dr. Lovett at 86 Kooyong Road, Armadale, Victoria, 3242, Australia.

On the horizon is pressure to introduce an experimental chicken pox vaccine for mass use. Members of a Federal Drug Administration (FDA) advisory committee are urging the FDA to approve a vaccine developed a decade ago and containing a live but weakened form of the varicella zoster virus—the first vaccine designed to produce a lifelong "silent infection" in the body. The vaccine's side effects (including shingles), level of effectiveness (study results vary), and duration of effectiveness are all under question. Several decades of use among children could, in the instance of short-term effectiveness, shift the disease to the adult population, where it is much more serious. The advisory board is reportedly requesting FDA approval and widescale safety and effectiveness studies if the vaccine is approved. (*Vaccine News*, p. 90)

In the past eight years alone, the full set of FDA-approved childhood vaccines has increased in scope and in price. In 1982, public health clinics were charging $6.69 to fully vaccinate a child against measles, mumps, rubella, polio, diphtheria, pertussis, and tetanus. Now, with the addition of a second measles dose and at least one Hib vaccine (to protect against meningitis), public health clinics are charging $91.20. ("Immunizations: Protecting Our Children," AAP memorandum, July 1990)

Ellen Kleiner

Good News

MORE VACCINE UPDATE

Dear *Mothering,*

In response to "Vaccine Updates" in Good News (Fall 1990), I want to share with readers the following information from *The Principles and Practice of Infectious Diseases,* a medical reference book edited by Drs. Mandell, Douglas, and Bennett (John Wiley & Sons, 1985).

Regarding measles vaccine: "Properly administered live measles vaccine has been associated with persistence of measles antibody for up to 15 years after vaccination."

Regarding mumps vaccine: "Although the antibody levels produced are lower than after natural infection, satisfactory titers are maintained for at least 10.5 years after vaccination."

Regarding rubella vaccine: "Rubella reinfection some months or years after receipt of rubella vaccine has also been observed . . . in up to 80% of persons who had received rubella vaccine previously and who were subsequently exposed to rubella during an epidemic. Reinfections have been more common in vaccinees than in those who had natural rubella. . . . It was at one time hoped that large numbers of immune people in a community could prevent rubella epidemics from occurring, so-called herd immunity. However, it has been documented that herd immunity does not decrease the spread of rubella. The question has been raised whether the antibody titer years after vaccination will remain high enough to prevent clinical rubella. Only time and continued surveillance will provide an answer to this question, but should antibody titers fall significantly, a booster vaccination could be given if necessary."

Regarding pertussis (whooping cough): "The marked reduction in the number of cases in recent years has been attributed to the availability and widespread use of pertussis vaccines. However, there was a decline in both incidence and mortality before general use of vaccine, suggesting that other factors may also be operating. . . . The presently available pertussis vaccines . . . do not confer either complete or permanent immunity. . . . Data suggest that although present vaccines are useful, improvements are needed if optimal protection of long duration is to be provided."

Regarding varicella-zoster virus (chicken pox): "Varicella is a relatively mild illness in normal children. There appears to be no urgency to develop a vaccine for universal use. . . . Widespread immunization . . . might lead to a change in the epidemiology of the disease so a larger number of older persons might be affected. One of the major objections to a live vaccine is the tendency of the virus to establish a latent infection. We would have to be certain that vaccine virus would not produce zoster more frequently or in a more severe form than the natural disease."

After reading this information one hardly wonders why high school and college students have been getting measles; why some states now require college students to show immunity to measles, mumps, and rubella; and why health officials focusing on measles have enacted what amounts to an adult vaccination law, as well as a two-dose requirement. Will health commissioners soon be telling us that four or five measles "boosters" are not only required but necessary to avoid the by then life-threatening possibility of getting the disease?

As for chicken pox, health officials are currently planning a mass vaccination requirement. In light of the above concerns with the chicken pox vaccine, our job is to organize *now* and let our federal and state legislators know that enough is enough. It is my hope that *Mothering* readers will write letters to the editors of their local newspapers, visit their federal and state legislators, talk to family and friends, and help prevent the passage of a chicken pox vaccine require-ment. When lots of voices are heard continuously, lawmakers pay attention.

The researchers' concerns about the chicken pox vaccine reflect what appears to have happened with the measles, mumps, and rubella vaccines; yet, instead of reevaluating immunization policy and possibly even recommending against vaccines, health policy officials are forging ahead with a new one.

Bonnie Plumeri Franz
Ogdensburg, New York

VACCINES IN THE TROPICS?

Dear *Mothering*,

My husband, 10-month-old son, and I have recently moved back to Guatemala to live on our farm. I've been searching for information on the different tropical diseases here—specifically, malaria, typhoid fever, and hepatitis A. We've decided not to give our baby the malaria prophylaxis, Chloroquine, after reading about the risks involved; he has taken it three times and vomited after each dose. He was also extremely sick after one typhoid vaccination, so we've opted against this inoculation, too. As for the hepatitis vaccine, it must be given every four months, which raises a number of questions.

Traditional doctors are in favor of all these medicines, but I would like to know what other families in tropical areas have done.

Sarah Lee
Izabal, Guatemala

VACCINATIONS AND INFORMED CHOICE

Magda Krance

Magda Krance is a freelance journalist whose work has appeared in Time, People, The New York Times, The Chicago Tribune, American Health, Par-enting, Spy, *and several other publications. She lives with her husband, Steve Leonard, and young son, Casimir, in Chicago, Illinois.*

My husband and I were uneasy as our son approached the age of two months, the time for his first diphtheria-pertussis-tetanus (DPT) shot. I had done extensive research on the subject of vaccinations the year before, and the tales of alleged adverse reactions to the pertussis component—brain damage, convulsions, physical handicaps, death—were horrifying, as were the suggestions that more subtle side effects, such as hyperactivity, learning disabilities, epilepsy, chronic allergies, asthma, vision and hearing problems, and even eczema might be linked to the inoculations. Additionally, the idea of someone injecting syringes full of toxoids and chemicals, including trace amounts of aluminum, formaldehyde (a mercury derivative), hydrochloric acid, and charcoal into our healthy son was disturbing.

Also distressing, though, was the newspaper article about the uninoculated children in a Buffalo, New York, family who came down with whooping cough, as pertussis is also known—a serious, sometimes fatal disease, especially for infants under six months of age. The violent coughing fits can cause babies to turn blue and to suffocate. *Uncomplicated* cases can last up to ten weeks, and hospitalization and intensive respiratory therapy are usually necessary. Although the children in the Buffalo family survived, the experience was no doubt as guilt provoking for the parents who had elected to forgo the shots as it was physically traumatic for the kids who had no say in the matter.

Of course, one seldom sees articles about the millions of children who have been vaccinated without incident, and the smaller number who have not had the shots but still remained healthy, or have become ill and recovered without complications. As frightening as the horror stories about children who have been injured by vaccines are, it is important to remember that they do not reflect the experience of the vast majority.

Generally, the risk of vaccine injury appears to be relatively low, although it is difficult to say exactly how low for several reasons: some possible pertussis reactions may be misdiagnosed as Sudden Infant Death Syndrome (SIDS); the reporting of vaccine injuries and the correlation of them to vaccine batch numbers have not been comprehensive over the years; and the manifestations of the alleged effects may occur after children have been exposed to other agents that cause similar problems, making it difficult for parents or medical professionals to connect, and especially to prove, cause and effect.

Even though *any* possibility of vaccine injury can be alarming to parents, it is essential to keep the inoculation controversy in perspective. Children are at far greater risk of accidental death every day in the bathtub or the family car than they are from becoming ill as a result of inoculations. Because most of the American population has been vaccinated, and because sanitation conditions are so much better than in previous times, the hazard of exposure is also very low.

Although it is not quite a Sophie's choice, still the decisions about inoculations that face parents can be agonizing. Because of societal pressures, parents sometimes feel that they have no choice at all, since proof of vaccination is required before children are admitted to schools, and this often applies to daycare centers as well. We want to take it on faith that vaccinations are safe; the idea, after all, is to protect our children, not to harm them. Besides, most of us got the full battery of obligatory inoculations when we were children, and most of us turned out fine. Moreover, although most of us born before the measles-mumps-rubella vaccine was developed got itchy or chipmunk-cheeked, we also received sympathy and attention, and got to stay in bed and watch TV. For the most part those childhood illnesses seemed like a tolerable rite of passage, at least in the clean, comfortable circumstances of my home. In impoverished, unsanitary settings, though, they can be lethal.

In recent years, there have been several outbreaks of measles and whooping cough around the country. These incidents have been accompanied by urgent drives for universal vaccination, warnings of the dire consequences of exposure to the diseases, and reassurances that studies have conclusively shown the pertussis vaccine to be safe. At the same time, dozens of heartrending stories about children who have been allegedly injured by vaccines (as well as their heartbroken, financially ruined parents) have appeared on television and in consumer publications over the past decade, causing increasing numbers of parents, and even some medical professionals, to question the safety of the pertussis vaccine and the wisdom of mandatory vaccination programs (which have been canceled in most Western European countries).

Currently both proponents and opponents of the pertussis vaccine are armed with arsenals of persuasive rhetoric and manipulated statistics. It is difficult to know which side to trust when the issue is as emotionally charged as your child's health and future. Should you trust the physicians and public health officials who insist that there is no proven link between the pertussis vaccine and brain damage, that the benefits of vaccination in general far outweigh the risks, that epidemics would sweep the country and harm vastly more children if the inoculations were not mandatory, that society's interests outweigh those of the individual, and that the few children who may be injured or killed by vaccines should be considered unfortunate but necessary "altruists"? Or should you trust those who oppose compulsory vaccination, who counter that some inoculations can cause injury and death, that they do not necessarily confer immunity (many of the teenagers who have gotten measles in the recent outbreaks had been vaccinated), and that they should be a matter of personal choice?

There are no easy answers. Informed choice and consent are essential to safeguard your child's health. Parents have to be smart health consumers. The best path to follow is to personally investigate the pros and cons of vaccination in the context of your child's own medical history. Know all the options and ramifications before you decide whether you want your child to have any, some, or all of the recommended vaccinations. Find out what each shot contains and what the risks are of both the disease and the inoculation. For detailed information on vaccine ingredients, side effects, and contraindications (conditions in which a vaccine should not be given), check in the *Physicians' Desk Reference* in the reference section of the library, or ask to see your pharmacist's copy. A useful source of information on infectious diseases is the American Academy of Pediatrics' (AAP) *Red Book*; ask to see your physician's copy during your next office visit.

Granted, it is not easy to be well informed; it takes persistence and time. Pamphlets promoting vaccination are ubiquitously available at schools and clinics, but information from those opposing vaccinations is more difficult to find. Concerned parents have to seek it out in medical reference books, in several books on the subject, and in newsletters and pamphlets distributed by ad hoc groups and alternative health organizations. If you only have time to read one book, read Harris L. Coulter and Barbara Loe Fisher's *DPT: A Shot in the Dark* (New York: Harcourt Brace Jovanovich, 1985), a remarkable work that blends personal stories with solid scientific research and reporting. Remember, however, that all information provided by either side has to be taken with a grain of salt.

Before making decisions regarding vaccinations, it may also be helpful to speak to people who have firsthand experience with the vaccines. Although their opinions will vary, they may provide a broader context in which to make judgments. Robert Daum, MD, professor of pediatrics and head of pediatric infectious diseases at the University of Chicago, and member of the AAP's committee on infectious diseases, approves of "consumer awareness and education regarding the effects and side effects of all medical interventions. It's wonderful to have parents who seek information about the interventions being offered to their children. You can get a parent working with you. But I am also strongly provaccine. I believe that preventive medicine saves great anguish and suffering from the diseases the vaccines are designed to prevent. Polio and smallpox are gone only because immunizations have gotten rid of them. Immunization is such an important preventive medicine strategy." He notes with alarm that because of increased reports of vaccine injuries, "the risk-benefit analysis as perceived by society has changed. With whooping cough, you have a disease that used to kill young babies, and you have a vaccine that for many years was perceived as safe. Then a television show does an exposé on DPT ["DPT Vaccine Roulette" was broadcast by NBC in 1982], and suddenly it's perceived as unsafe, the lawsuits go through the roof, and public acceptance of the vaccine goes down. I've seen the diseases, I've seen the burden, and I feel good about recommending immunizations."

As an example of the opposite viewpoint, Kathi Williams believes her learning-disabled son suffered an adverse reaction to his fourth DPT shot nine years ago—an event which coincided with the televising of "DPT Vaccine Roulette." She and others who called the station after seeing the program were put in touch with each other; they subsequently formed a support and watchdog group, Dissatisfied Parents Together (DPT), which lobbies for safer vaccination programs, and which now operates the National Vaccine Information Center (204-F Mill St., Vienna, VA 22180; 703-938-3783). "Our concern is that the AAP and CDC [Centers for Disease Control] want to prevent disease at all costs, the 'costs' being some children," says Williams. "It's a war on disease, but the 'soldiers' are the children. When it's your child, the risks are 100 percent—there are no benefits."

Thanks in part to intense lobbying by DPT and other groups concerned about the safety of the pertussis vaccine, the National Childhood Vaccine Injury Act passed in 1986 and was enacted in 1988. It requires doctors to record the batch, lot number, and date of all vaccines given, and to report adverse reactions to the CDC.

If you decide to have your child vaccinated, be sure to get a copy of the completed form for each injection from the doctor for your own records. You will need the information in the unlikely event that your child suffers an adverse reaction that should be reported, such as high fever (over 103°), acute diarrhea or vomiting, convulsions, seizures, extended high-pitched screaming, paralysis, unconsciousness, or death. In the past, there was no systematic recording or reporting of such reactions, making it virtually impossible for parents whose children had been allegedly injured or killed by vaccines to link the events in court.

Most pediatricians now give parents a checklist of possible side effects to watch for following the DPT inoculation, the vaccine with the highest rate of adverse reactions because of the pertussis component. If such a list is not offered, ask for it. According to the CDC, convulsions (with or without fever) and shock occur in one in 1,750 doses of vaccine given, and permanent neurological damage—retardation, paralysis, spasticity—occurs in one out of 310,000 doses. It is recommended that each child receive five doses of the vaccine before entering school, and up to 20 million doses of DPT vaccine are given in the United States each year.

"Recording data by 'immunization' is thoroughly illogical [because] incidence expressed in terms of shots does not correlate with incidence in terms of children," contend Harris L. Coulter and Barbara Loe Fisher in their book *DPT: A Shot in the Dark* (recently updated, reprinted, and available in paperback). "It is misleading to give results in terms of shots administered," say Coulter and Fisher. "It is not shots that run high fevers, develop convulsions, become mentally retarded, or die. This happens to children." The authors cite a 1978 to 1979 study of adverse reactions to the pertussis vaccine conducted by the University of California–Los Angeles and the Food and Drug Administration (FDA), reporting that of the 3.3 million children vaccinated every year in the United States, within 48 hours nearly 8,500 have convulsions, nearly 8,500 undergo collapse, and about 16,000 have episodes of high-pitched (encephalitic) screaming, which may indicate central nervous system irritation.

Some other good points to consider are made by J. Anthony Morris, PhD, a former government virologist who was fired in 1976 because he was critical of the swine flu vaccination program, which produced a large number of injuries and lawsuits, many still unsettled to this day. Morris remarks, "I'm all for inoculation programs for measles, mumps, and rubella, but I'm against placing faulty vaccines on the market. The early measles vaccines were clearly faulty; the current pertussis vaccine is clearly faulty and could be improved." (A safer pertussis vaccine has been in use for several years in Japan, but has yet to be approved for use in this country.)

Another problem, Morris says, is the premise and practice of mass inoculation:

When a vaccine is mandated, then not only do the manufacturers get careless, but the pediatrician administering the vaccine gets careless. When you have mass vaccination programs . . . carelessness comes into play, and you give a vaccine to a child who shouldn't receive it at that time because of illness. . . . Carelessness is almost inescapable in mass vaccination programs, where you're concerned with the benefit that society derives, not with what happens to the individual child. It's like the army, but it's children being hurt, not soldiers. I'm against mass inoculations.

Each child should be considered as an individual. If that were the case, you would reduce to an insignificant [level] the number of cases of brain damage and death from the DPT vaccine.

If you decide you do not want your child to receive some of the inoculations, ask your physician to write a medical exemption. Some will; others may refuse to treat your child at all unless you agree to all the shots. Find out what vaccinations your state requires; the requirements and exemptions vary from state to state. Some states accept a philosophical or "personal belief" exemption as well as a religious exemption. Religious exemptions are accepted in most states and are not necessarily restricted to members of "recognized" religions, such as Christian Scientists, Jehovah's Witnesses, and Seventh-Day Adventists, who typically do invoke the exemption. Check carefully with your own state health department for the latest legislative changes.

In addition to obtaining sufficient information, communication is important in determining the correct course of action regarding vaccination; to protect your child's health, two-way communication with your doctor is not a luxury but a necessity. Ask lots of questions, rather than blindly submitting to a pediatrician's authority, as so many people are conditioned to do. Do not let your doctor tell you that he or she knows what is best for your child without giving reasons for such decisions. Good doctors should have no problem with requests for explanations, but less competent ones may get defensive or angry. If that happens, find another doctor.

Physicians, too, have to ask questions, to be sure that each child's health and family medical history do not pose the risk of a serious adverse reaction. You want your pediatrician to ask, and you need to be able to answer, the following questions: Has the child been sick lately? Is there currently any infection or fever? Is there a history of convulsions or neurological illness in the family? A history of allergies in the family? A history of drug use that might cause neurological problems in the child, such as maternal cocaine use during pregnancy? Was the child premature or did the child have a low birth weight? Are there any immune system problems? Has the child shown an allergic reaction to milk? Was there any cerebral irritation or injury at birth? Has the child had a bad reaction to a previous inoculation?

Unfortunately, such communication with doctors is sometimes difficult because families may be forced by HMOs to abruptly change care-givers, others are dependent on overcrowded public clinics, and physicians are pressured by too many patients and too little time. Consequently, it can be hard to make sure your pediatrician knows that your baby is just getting over a cold, or that epilepsy runs in the family, or whatever the mitigating factors may be.

I was braced for a disagreement with our baby's doctor when we took him in for his two-month exam. Before I could open my mouth, though, she announced, "I don't want to give him the pertussis component, because of the seizure he had after he was born." Indeed, he had had focal seizures in one hand when he was less than a day old, and had spent the next few days in intensive care until it was determined that my long labor had caused a tiny hemmorhage to form under his skull. Our pediatrician had made the correct decision regarding the pertussis vaccine, considering our baby's short but dramatic medical history. We were greatly relieved, and our child suffered no ill effects from the diphtheria-tetanus shot he received.

At present our knowledge about the effectiveness and dangers of vaccines is also being revised according to new data, some of which can be confusing. Although the medical community uses the words *inoculation, vaccination,* and *immunization* interchangeably, with *immunization* the favored term, vaccinations given to older children and young adults have not necessarily guaranteed immunity. In Houston, where 1,743 cases of measles were confirmed between October 1988 and June 1989, more than 50 percent of the cases were considered unpreventable, even though most in that group had been previously "immunized."

It is also advisable to be current regarding the latest information about the effectiveness of various vaccines, since that information is updated and revised according to new medical research and the experiences of those who have been vaccinated. For example, the measles vaccine administered during the 1970s lacked a stabilizer, and consequently lost its efficacy if left unrefrigerated; a stabilizer was not added until 1980. Another example is the fact that until the mid-1970s, babies were vaccinated against measles between the ages of 9 and 12 months. However, subsequently it was discovered that maternal antibodies in the baby interfered with the vaccine's effectiveness, which is why the measles shot is now administered to children when they are 15 months old.

My pediatrician's office recently faxed me several pages of information from the AAP's *Red Book* about pertussis symptoms and treatment. Included was the estimate that vaccine efficacy for young children who have received at least three doses of DPT vaccine is 80 percent. The report also said that vaccine-induced "immunity" lasts for about three years, and then gradually diminishes. Does that mean that 20 percent of vaccinated children may come down with whooping cough, if they are exposed? Does it mean that all vaccinated individuals have a 20 percent chance of getting whooping cough? And if so, does it still make sense to vaccinate?

Probably not, says Richard Moskowitz, MD, a conventionally trained family practitioner who now practices homeopathic medicine in the Boston area. Moskowitz believes that evolution has produced a hardy immune system, "the normal maturation of which requires the ability to mount and recover from a strong acute illness, such as the measles. By programming our children [through inoculation] to respond chronically rather than acutely, we retard the development of the immune system," he maintains. "If what the vaccines did was to confer a true immunity similar to what you receive when you get and recover from the measles, then the unvaccinated children would be at risk only to themselves. The extent to which they're a risk to others is a very precise measurement of the inefficacy of the vaccine."

Although physicians may disagree about the effectiveness of various vaccines, many agree that the question of whether or not to inoculate children should be the parents' choice. Moskowitz admits he has more "persistent and troubling" questions than answers about vaccination, and for that reason, says he has "a lot of difficulty recommending compulsory vaccinations to people against their will. If people want the vaccinations, I have no problem with that. That's their right. But I think parents should have the choice."

Anthony Morris, too, thinks parents should have the final say. "It's not necessary to mandate a program whose benefits are overwhelming," he says. "Logistically, it's easier to carry out mandatory inoculations, but democracy is not supposed to be easy. If you give a parent all the facts about the benefits and risks of vaccination, then the parent will make a wise choice. The parent will almost invariably say yes to vaccination voluntarily."

IMMUNIZATIONS

Risks and rates of diseases, risks and rates of side effects of recommended vaccinations. (Courtesy of Centers for Disease Control, Atlanta)

Disease/
Number of reported cases
in United States in 1988:

Symptoms/mortality rate

Diphtheria/1

Can cause infection in nose, throat, and skin; can interfere with breathing; sometimes causes heart failure or paralysis. 1:10 die from it in the United States.

Pertussis/3,008

Also called whooping cough; causes severe coughing spells that can interfere with eating, drinking, and breathing. In the United States, 70 percent of reported cases occur in children under five years of age; more than 50 percent of those under one year of age are hospitalized. In the United States, 1:4 children with pertussis develop pneumonia. 22:1,000 develop convulsions and/or other brain problems. An average of nine deaths a year are caused by pertussis in the United States.

Tetanus/49	Also called lockjaw; results when wounds are infected with tetanus bacteria, which are often found in dirt. If the wound is not properly cleaned, a poison forms in the wound and causes muscle spasms. In the United States, 4:10 who get tetanus die from it.
*Measles/3,643	Usually causes rash, high fever, cough, runny nose, watery eyes for one to two weeks. Can be more serious: causes ear infection or pneumonia in 1:10 children who get it; causes encephalitis in 1:1,000 children who get it, which can lead to convulsions, deafness, or mental retardation. 2:10,000 children who contract measles die from it.
Mumps/4,730	Usually produces fever, headache, and inflammation of salivary glands, causing cheeks to swell. Can be more serious, resulting in mild meningitis in 1:10 children. More rarely, can cause deafness or enccphalitis. In adolescent or adult males who get mumps, 1:4 can develop painful inflammation of the testicles, causing sterility in rare cases.
Rubella/221	Also called German measles. Usually very

mild, causing slight fever, rash, and swelling of neck glands. Lasts about three days. In adult women, may cause joint swelling for one to two weeks. Very rarely, can cause encephalitis or purpura (temporary bleeding disorder). In pregnant women, can cause miscarriage or birth defects.

Polio/2   Virus disease that can cause permanent crippling and occasionally death.

Note: the CDC does not have data on how many of these individuals were vaccinated and came down with the disease anyway.

*According to George Seastrom of the CDC's Immunizations Division, as of 25 June 1989 there was a 370 percent increase in measles cases over the 1988 total. As of that date there were 7,022 cases of measles reported, as opposed to 1,492 cases reported the previous year at the same time.

The 7,022 measles cases break down as follows:

Preschoolers:	3,553
School age (K–12):	1,367
College age:	365
Other:	779

According to the CDC's Seastrom, "of school-age children, over 90 percent have been adequately vaccinated. As far as preschoolers are concerned, depending on the area of the country, it would range from 40 to 60 percent." The percentages reflect the fact that some parents may not take their children in for inoculations until they are required to do so, when the children are ready to enter school. (Many daycare centers and preschools also require proof of immunization before admitting children.) According to Samuel Katz of Duke University's School of Medicine, there is a drop in the numbers of children being immunized, because their parents were not yet born during the prevaccine epidemics, and are thus unaware of the dangers.

Vaccines(s)	Rate of protection/side effects/ rate of occurrence/contraindications
DPT/DT/Td (diphtheria-pertussis-tetanus)	More than 95 percent of those who receive the full series of shots are protected from tetanus. Diphtheria and pertussis parts of the vaccine are not as effective, but still protect most children from getting the disease, and make the disease milder for those who do get it.

With DPT vaccine, most children will have a slight fever and be irritable within two days of inoculation. Half will have some soreness and swelling in the shot area. In 1:330 shots, a temperature of 105° or more may occur. In 1:100 shots, continuous crying for three or more hours may result. In 1:900 shots, unusual high-pitched crying may occur. In 1:1,750 cases, convulsions, limpness, or paleness may be caused by the shot. In 1:10,000 shots, severe brain problems may occur, and in 1:310,000 shots, permanent brain damage may result. These side effects are caused by the pertussis component of the shot; DT or Td shots may cause soreness and slight fever.

Children who have had a serious reaction to a DPT shot should not receive additional pertussis vaccine. Children who have previously had a convulsion or are suspected of having any nervous system problem should not receive DPT vaccine without thorough medical evaluation; likewise if there is any family history of convulsions or nervous system problems. Children who are currently sick should not receive DPT until they are well. And children undergoing treatment that may lower resistance to infection (e.g., cortisone, prednisone, radiation therapy, and so forth) should not receive DPT.

MMR
(measles, mumps,
rubella)

About 90 percent of those who are inoculated will have protection, probably for life, if not vaccinated before the age of 15 months. 1:5 children will get a rash or slight fever lasting a few days one to two weeks after receiving the measles vaccine. Occasionally, there may be mild swelling of salivary glands caused by the mumps vaccine. 1:7 children will get a rash or some swelling of neck glands one or two weeks after getting rubella vaccine. 1:20 children will have some aching or swelling of joints one to three weeks after receiving rubella vaccine, lasting a few days. In adults, 4:10 may have temporary joint swelling after rubella vaccine; 2:100 may develop true arthritis after the vaccine. Very rarely, children may develop encephalitis, convulsions with fever, and neurological problems after the MMR vaccinations.

Anyone who is currently sick should not have the MMR shot until healthy. Anyone who has had a severe allergic reaction to eating eggs should not take the measles or mumps components. Anyone with cancer, leukemia, or lymphoma should not take the shot. Nor should anyone taking medication that reduces resistance to infection.

OPV (oral polio vaccine)

In more than 90 percent of those inoculated, OPV gives long-term, possibly lifelong protection. 1:8,100,000 doses of OPV causes paralytic polio in the person vaccinated. 1:5,000,000 doses may cause paralytic polio in a close contact of a recently vaccinated person.

OPV should not be taken by anyone with cancer, leukemia, or lymphoma; by anyone taking medication that reduces resistance to infection; by anyone living in the same household with anyone who has any of the above conditions; by anyone who is currently sick; or by pregnant women. Anyone over the age of 18 should avoid inoculation unless there is an outbreak in the community.

IPV (injectable polio vaccine)

Also called killed polio vaccine; it has no known risk of causing paralytic polio. IPV is recommended for persons with low resistance to serious infections, or for those living with persons with low resistance. It may also be recommended for previously unvaccinated adults whose children are to be vaccinated with OPV.

Magda Krance

Mothering, no. 63 Spring 1992

THE MMR VACCINE

Lynne McTaggart

Lynne McTaggart is an award-winning investigative journalist, author of several books, and editor of the newsletter What Doctors Don't Tell You. She lives in London, England, with her husband Bryan and their daughter Caitlin. "The MMR Vaccine" first appeared in Mothering, no. 63 (Spring 1992).

My two-year-old daughter Caitlin and I are the targets of a £1.5 million ($2.7 million) advertising campaign. The British government and even my local health clinic are attempting to convince me to have her vaccinated against measles, mumps, and rubella (German measles).

Traditionally, the MMR campaign was restricted to physician handouts—brochures stating that the vaccine has for many years been used safely in other countries, particularly the United States, and that it provides "lifelong protection against all three infections with a single jab." Now, emotive messages of all sorts are appearing in television ads depicting angelic sleeping children.

Parents in the United States are under similar pressure to give their children the live triple vaccine. The United States government has suggested withholding welfare payments from any mother refusing to vaccinate her child. And Chicago health authorities have begun using loudspeaker sales pitches mixed with salsa music to encourage Hispanic mothers to take their children to neighborhood health clinics for shots.

A Spotty Take-Up Record

The recent fuss has come precisely because the vaccine appears not to be working. The United States is witnessing a steadily increasing epidemic of measles—the worst in decades—even though the combined shot has been available since 1975, and the measles vaccine itself has been in effect since 1957. While the government-targeted date for elimination of the disease was set at 1982, the Centers for Disease Control (CDC) in Atlanta reported a provisional total of 27,672 cases of measles in 1990.

This figure represents twice the amount reported in 1989, which was twice that reported in 1988.[1]

At first, the measles vaccine looked promising. The number of measles cases fell by 25 percent to 63,000 the year it was introduced. After bottoming out at 1,500 in 1983, though, the number of cases swelled 423 percent by 1989, and is now sharply rising, especially in Houston, Texas, and Los Angeles County.[2]

The medical establishment blames the recent epidemic on clusters of unvaccinated children, especially those in poor, nonwhite neighborhoods. Statistics, however, prove otherwise. CDC data from 1989 show that half of all college-age victims had been vaccinated. Moreover, between 1985 and 1986, two-thirds of all measles cases occurred in school-age children, the majority of whom had been vaccinated.[3]

"The appearance of measles is a sensitive indicator of the inadequacies of our vaccination system," announced Donald A. Henderson, chair of the National Vaccine Advisory Committee of the US Department of Health and Human Services, in tacit admission of the vaccine's failure. "It raises the specter of whether we might expect further down the line outbreaks of polio (should it be imported), pertussis and diphtheria."[4]

The epidemics occurring among college-age students are primarily affecting those born between 1957 and 1967, when the measles vaccine was introduced. The CDC currently estimates that between 5 and 15 percent of college students are susceptible.[5] As a result, students at many universities must provide proof of recent vaccination before registering for classes.

The problem, say CDC and other medical experts, is that the

vaccine wears off in time, as does an individual's immunity. Others believe that those vaccinated between 1957 and 1980 received a less stable version of the vaccine than those who were vaccinated more recently. Consequently, experts in the United States and elsewhere are recommending a variety of approaches: lowering the age of vaccination from 15 months to one year, or providing a measles booster shot at school age or later (around age 11) if the earlier booster has not been given, or administering the single measles shot at 9 months and the combined shot at 15 months, or introducing the MMR at one year of age.

The American Academy of Pediatrics now recommends giving a second dose of MMR at age two. Still, some medics believe that not even two doses will be enough to deal with the "wild" strains of measles that have been appearing. Underlying all these "solutions" is the disquieting question: *Does it make sense to offer booster shots of any sort if a single shot of the vaccine has not been shown to do the job?*

Theories on vaccine ineffectiveness abound. According to some, shots are given too early, and their effectiveness is canceled out by maternal antibodies acquired in the womb. Others imply that the vaccine loses its potency if given when children have respiratory infections, or if the serum is improperly stored or handled.

The CDC estimates that up to 10 percent of all vaccinations do not take.[6] And indeed, study after study points unerringly to clusters of vaccinated children who have contracted measles. Here are just a few examples:

■ In a 1986 outbreak of measles in Corpus Christi, Texas, 99 percent of the children had been vaccinated and more than 95 percent were purportedly immune.[7]

■ In 1987, the CDC reported 2,440 cases of measles among vaccinated children. Forty-one percent of them had received the MMR vaccine between 12 and 14 months of age, and the remaining 59 percent had been vaccinated at 15 months or older.[8]

■ In 1985, 80 percent of all cases of measles in the United States occurred in children who had been properly vaccinated at the appropriate age.[9]

■ Between 1985 and 1986, reports of measles outbreaks among school-age children revealed that 60 percent of them had been vaccinated.[10]

The rubella component of the vaccine has not fared well either. In the 1970s, Stanley Plotkin, MD, a professor of pediatrics at the University of Pennsylvania, evaluated adolescent girls who had received the vaccine during childhood. He found that more than one-third of them lacked any evidence of immunity against rubella.[11] More recently, an Italian study of 600 vaccinated girls showed that 10 percent of them had been infected by a wild strain of the virus—some within a few years of inoculation.[12]

Disease-Related Complications

The medical justification for the shots is that measles is a dangerous disease. Official statistics suggest that between 1 in 1,000 and 1 in 5,000 children who contract measles naturally—that is, not in response to the vaccine—will develop acute encephalitis (inflammation of the brain). Several years later, 1 in 5,000 of these youngsters will develop subacute sclerosing panencephalitis (SSPE), an often fatal progressive disease that causes hardening of the brain.[13]

The SSPE Registry report on the incidence of SSPE between 1960 and 1970, however, states that the measles-induced form of this disease is "very rare," occurring in 1 per million cases.[14] Furthermore, a study of 52 people with SSPE concludes that environmental factors other than measles, such as serious head injuries or close exposure to certain animals, contributed to the onset of disease. Researchers found "no differences with regard to the average age at vaccination, having received more than one measles vaccination, or having received measles vaccine after natural measles."[15]

Of the 89 suspected measles-associated deaths in the United States in 1990, most occurred in low-income populations. Inadequate nutrition and poor living conditions played a part in the outcome, as did failure to treat complications.[16]

Childhood mumps and rubella, on the other hand, are ordinarily very mild illnesses, says Dr. Norman Begg, consultant epidemiologist with the Public Health Laboratory Service, which recommended the triple vaccine in Britain. Mumps "very rarely" leads to long-term permanent complications, he notes. "On its own, mumps isn't a particularly cost-effective vaccine. But it provides extra benefit for the combined MMR vaccine."[17]

Vaccine-Related Complications

Risks are inherent in the vaccines themselves, and these appear far greater than the medical establishment claims. Moreover, complications are multiplied by a triple jab whose separate components carry individual risks.

According to the prevailing medical view, measles-vaccine-induced encephalitis is rare, occurring in 1 out of 200,000 children. Symptoms include fever, headache, possible convulsions, and behavioral changes. "Most symptoms are mild," says Begg, "and the children will recover."[18] The reported incidence of mumps-vaccine-induced meningitis is between 1 per 50,000 and 1 per million doses.[19]

Some studies using the same vaccine strains reveal significantly larger risks. A West German study places the incidence of reactions to the measles portion of the shot at 1 neurologic complication per 2,500 vaccinees and 1 case of temporary encephalitis per 17,650 vaccinees.[20] In several more recent studies, the measles vaccine strain recovered from victims' spines shows conclusively that the vaccine caused the encephalitis, says Dr. J. Anthony Morris, an immunization specialist formerly with the National Institutes of Health and the Food and Drug Administration.[21]

Of the first 10,000 British children given the measles vaccine, 2.5 per 1,000 suffered convulsions.[22] Wellcome, until recently one of three manufacturers of the MMR vaccine in Britain, reports that the measles portion of the vaccine may cause fever and rash, orchitis (inflammation of the testicle), nerve deafness, febrile convulsions, encephalitis, Guillain-Barré syndrome (a form of paralysis), SSPE, and atypical measles (marked by unusual symptoms).[23] In fact, the SSPE study cited above indicates that nearly one-third of all victims had received a measles vaccine prior to the onset of illness. "This study cannot confirm or rule out the possibility that the measles vaccine may lead to SSPE on rare occasions," conclude the authors.[24]

The mumps vaccine, too, is associated with complications. It is known to cause encephalitis, meningitis, seizures, unilateral nerve deafness, and other serious conditions. Researchers investigating all cases of mumps encephalitis over the previous 15 years concluded that one-sixth of them were due to the vaccine. "A recent increase appeared to be related to the introduction of a new mumps vaccine," they noted.[25] A Canadian study set the risk of mumps-vaccine-induced encephalitis at 1 per 100,000 recipients;[26] a Yugoslavian study, at 1 per 1,000 recipients.[27]

Several physicians have written letters to *The Lancet* describing reactions to the mumps portion of the MMR vaccine. An Edinburgh doctor reported that a girl who had developed meningitis 21 days after the shot had the mumps virus strain isolated from her spinal fluid, and it matched the strain used in the vaccine.[28] A West German doctor wrote in to say that health authorities in his country had come up with 27 neurological reactions to this component of the shot, including meningitis, febrile convulsions, encephalitis, and epilepsy.[29]

According to Wellcome, the rubella portion of the vaccine causes arthritis in 3 percent of child vaccinees and 12 to 20 percent of adult women recipients. "Symptoms may persist for a matter of months or, on rare occasions, for years," the company reports; and effects range from mild aches in the joints to extreme crippling.[30]

Robert Mendelsohn, MD, in reporting on the work of Aubrey Tingle, MD—a pediatric immunologist at Children's Hospital in Vancouver, British Columbia—points out that 30 percent of adults exposed to rubella vaccine developed arthritis two to four weeks afterward. Tingle also found the rubella virus in one-third of all adults and children with rheumatoid arthritis.[31]

This jibes with a 1970 Department of Health, Education and Welfare report citing that as many as "26 percent of children receiving rubella vaccination in national testing programs developed arthralgia and arthritis. Many had to seek medical attention, and some were hospitalized to test for rheumatic fever and rheumatoid arthritis."[32]

Morris testified against these and other vaccines in congressional hearings and, in the process, paved the way for the National Childhood Vaccine Injury Act that now awards remuneration to victims of vaccines. In his view, all statistics thus far published on side effects of the triple jab are extremely conservative. "We only hear about the encephalitis and the deaths," he says. "But there is an entire spectrum of reactions between fever and death, and it's all those things in between that never get reported."[33]

Part of that spectrum involves the temporary or imperfect immunity conferred by the vaccine. Many vaccinated children, for example, may grow up susceptible to measles, mumps, or rubella—each of which is far more serious, even deadly, in adulthood. Ample evidence already indicates that vaccinated children can contract new diseases such as atypical measles, which is more serious than the ordinary variety, often causing pneumonia and severe pain.[34]

Of special concern is the high failure rate of the rubella portion of the shot—sometimes within only five years of vaccination. This part of the vaccine was designed to eliminate German measles not so much in young children, but among women of childbearing age. The hope was to counteract the likelihood of contracting the disease while pregnant and thus bearing a child with possible birth defects. The vaccine, however, wears off; and when it does, one becomes susceptible to German measles. *In fact, vaccinated populations of women are more likely to contract the illness during pregnancy than are those who had German measles naturally in childhood, because the illness itself tends to confer lifelong immunity.*

Toward True Immunity

How I would love to get my hands on a magic bullet that would wipe out in an instant all the feverish, sleepless nights my little one may have to suffer as she struggles through the various childhood illnesses—for the battle, I've decided, is the best option there is. The vaccine presently on offer is simply too experimental, too ineffective, and too risky; and the illnesses it is designed to prevent are rarely life threatening to healthy, well-nourished children, especially those who've been breastfed.

Even when the most serious of these illnesses strikes, less drastic health measures are available. *The Lancet* recently reported that giving vitamin A to children with severe measles lessens the complications of illness and the chances of dying. Indeed, author Gerald T. Keusch, MD, of Boston's New England Medical Center, concluded that children benefit from appropriate doses of vitamin A whenever they exhibit a vitamin A deficiency or even the possibility of complications due to measles.[35]

Two of Caitlin's unvaccinated friends recently came down with measles. Their reactions were mild, a bit like the flu. Now they will have true immunity to measles for the rest of their lives. I am putting my money where their mothers put theirs: on nature's own tried-and-tested immunization program.

Notes

1. "Measles: United States, 1990," *Journal of the American Medical Association* (26 June 1991): 3227.

2. William K. Stevens, "Despite Vaccine, Perilous Measles Won't Go Away," *The New York Times* (14 March 1989): C–6.

3. "Measles Immunization: Recommendations, Challenges and More Information" (editorial), *Journal of the American Medical Association* (24 April 1991): 2111.

4. "Secretary of Health, Human Services to Hear Recommendations for Improving Immunization," *Journal of the American Medical Association* (17 October 1990): 1925.

5. "Campus Ills," *Time* Magazine (11 March 1985): 66.

6. "Measles Prevention: Supplementary Statement," *Journal of the American Medical Association* (10 February 1989): 827.

7. Tracy L. Gustafson et al., "Measles Outbreak in a Fully Immunized Secondary School Population," *New England Journal of Medicine* (26 March 1987): 771–774.

8. "Measles in the USA," *The Pediatric Infectious Disease Journal Newsletter* (September 1987): 18.

9. *Morbidity and Mortality Weekly Report* (6 June 1987); cited in Robert S. Mendelsohn, *But Doctor . . . About That Shot* (Chicago, IL: The People's Doctor, 1988), p. 81.

10. Laurie E. Markowitz et al., "Patterns of Transmission in Measles Outbreaks in the United States: 1985–6," *New England Journal of Medicine* (12 January 1989): 75.

11. See Note 9, p. 21.

12. M. G. Cusi et al. (correspondence), *The Lancet* (27 October 1990): 1070.

13. David Isaacs and Margaret Menser, "Modern Vaccines: Measles, Mumps, Rubella, and Varicella," *The Lancet* (27 October 1990): 1385.

14. J. T. Jabbour et al., "Epidemiology of Subacute Sclerosing Panencephalitis (SSPE)," *Journal of the American Medical Association* (15 May 1972): 959.

15. Neal A. Halsey et al., "Risk Factors in Subacute Sclerosing Panencephalitis: A Case Control Study," *Journal of the American Medical Association* (4 November 1980): 415–424.

16. New York Times News Service.

17. Dr. Norman Begg, in an interview with the author (December 1989).

18. Ibid.

19. See Note 13, p. 1385.

20. H. Allerdist, "Neurological Complications Following Measles Vaccination"; presented at the International Symposium on Immunization: Benefit versus Risk Factors, in Brussels (1978); published in *Development of Biological Standards 432* (1979): 259–264.

21. Dr. J. Anthony Morris, in an interview with the author (December 1989).

22. "Mumps, Meningitis and MMR Vaccination" (editorial), *The Lancet* (28 October 1989): 1016.

23. *ABPI Data Sheet Compendium, 1989–90* (London, England: Datapharm Publications, 1989), p. 1717.

24. See Note 15, pp. 417–421.

25. Jane McDonald et al., "Clinical and Epidemiological Features of Mumps Meningoencephalitis and Possible Vaccine-Related Disease," *Pediatric Infectious Disease Journal* (November 1989): 751–754.

26. See Note 22, p. 1017.

27. Milan Cizman et al., "Aseptic Meningitis after Vaccination against Measles and Mumps," *Pediatric Infectious Disease Journal* (May 1989): 302.

28. James A. Gray and Sheila M. Burns (correspondence), *The Lancet* (14 October 1989): 98.

29. W. Ehrengut (correspondence), *The Lancet* (23 September 1989): p. 751.

30. See Note 23, p. 1718.

31. See Note 9, p. 30.

32. *Science* (26 March 1977); cited in Walene James, *Immunization: The Reality behind the Myth* (Hadley, MA: Bergin & Garvey, 1988), p. 12.

33. Dr. J. Anthony Morris, in an interview with the author (January 1990).

34. Z. Spirer et al. (correspondence), *Pediatric Infectious Disease Journal* (March 1986): 276–277.

35. Gerald T. Keusch, "Vitamin A Supplements—Too Good Not to Be True," *New England Journal of Medicine* (4 October 1990): 985–987.

VACCINATION: A SACRAMENT OF MODERN MEDICINE

Adapted from a lecture given by Richard Moskowitz

Richard Moskowitz, MD, received his undergraduate degree from Harvard University and his medical degree from New York University before studying homeopathy with George Vithoulkas in Athens, Greece. He recently served as president of the National Center for Homeopathy in Washington, DC, and is the author of a book on homeopathy in pregnancy and birth to be published in 1993 by North Atlantic Press. A Contributing Editor to Mothering, *Dr. Moskowitz currently practices classical homeopathy in Watertown, Massachusetts. "Vaccination: A Sacrament of Modern Medicine" first appeared in* Mothering, *no. 63 (Spring 1992).*

In Western medicine, vaccines have become sacraments of our faith in biotechnology. By that I mean, first, that their efficacy and safety are widely seen as self-evident and needing no further proof; second, that they are given routinely to all children, by force if necessary, in the interest of the public good; and finally, that they ritually initiate our loyal participation in the medical enterprise as a whole. Vaccines celebrate our right and power as a civilization to manipulate biological processes *ad libitum* (and for profit), without undue concern for or even an explicit concept of the total health of populations about to be subjected to them.

These special privileges give some measure of the reverence accorded to vaccines in what can only be called the religion of modern medicine.[1] Its theology, as practiced in the United States and to some extent throughout the developed world, involves glaring inconsistencies such as minimal standards of vaccine effectiveness that disregard the total health of the organism; enforcement of compulsory vaccination laws in the absence of any obvious public health emergency; and suspension of the normal rules of scientific inquiry in their honor.

The Measles Vaccine

I would like to begin with a brief history of the measles vaccine, which illustrates many issues pertaining to the other vaccines as well. In its natural state, the measles virus enters the body of a susceptible person through the nose and mouth, and incubates silently for about 14 days in the lymphoid tissues of the nasopharynx, the regional lymph nodes, and finally the liver, spleen, bone marrow, and lymphocytes and macrophages of the peripheral blood. The illness known as measles is the process by which the virus is expelled from the blood through the nose and mouth, the same orifices through which it entered. This massive, concerted outpouring of the entire immune system culminates in the targeting of the virus by specific antibodies, and the ability to synthesize them on short notice remains encoded as a permanent "memory" of the experience—a virtual guarantee that people who have recovered from measles will *never* get it again, no matter how many times they are reexposed.

In addition to conferring lifelong immunity against the measles virus, the natural recovery process "primes" the organism to respond promptly and efficiently to other microorganisms in the future. Indeed, the ability to mount a vigorous, acute response to infection deserves recognition as being indispensable to the maturation of a healthy immune system.

Measles is about 20 percent fatal in populations exposed to it for the first time. In the United States and many other countries, centuries of adaptation and "herd immunity" have slowly and painfully transformed it into an ordinary childhood disease with nonspecific mechanisms in place to help deal with it effectively. The permanent immunity acquired in recovering from the natural disease thus represents a net gain for the total health of the human race.

"True" or lifelong immunity of this type cannot be ascribed to the measles vaccine. In contrast to the natural disease, the vaccine virus produces no local sensitization at the portal of entry, no incubation, no massive outpouring, and no acute disease. It can elicit long-term antibody production only by surviving in latent form in the lymphocytes and macrophages of the blood.

Because the vaccinated individual has no obvious way of getting rid of the virus, the technical feat of antibody synthesis presumably represents, at most, a memory of *chronic infection.*

It makes no sense to claim that vaccines render us "immune" to viruses if in fact they weaken our ability to expel them and force us to harbor them permanently. Indeed, my concern and growing conviction is that such a carrier state tends to compromise our ability to respond to other infections as well. In that sense, vaccines must themselves be regarded as immuno-suppressive.

In the United States, the laws mandating vaccination against measles were enacted in the early 1960s, when the disease was limited almost entirely to elementary schoolchildren and both deaths and serious complications were at an all-time low. With vaccination rates soon exceeding 95 percent in most states, the incidence of measles throughout the country dropped from the prevaccine era average of over 400,000 cases annually to less than 5,000 cases in the early 1980s.[2] It looked as though the disease would soon be eliminated.

In the 1980s, however, the almost universal faith in vaccinations began to unravel. Measles started reappearing in even fully vaccinated populations, and public health authorities began grappling with the mysterious phenomenon of "vaccine failure."

In 1984, 27 cases of measles were reported at a high school in Waltham, Massachusetts, where over 98 percent of the students had documentary proof of vaccination.[3] In 1989, an Illinois high school with vaccination records on 99.7 percent of its students reported 69 cases over a three-week period.[4] These reports failed to mention the surprisingly low number of measles cases appearing in unvaccinated students. Still, the published data strongly contradicted official claims of a "reservoir" of the disease among the unvaccinated, a mythology used both then and now to frighten wavering parents into compliance.

The data from various outbreaks indicated a resurgence of the disease mainly in older children and adolescents, groups with the highest rates of serious complications. Health officials dutifully suggested that vaccine-mediated "immunity" was only temporary and wore off with increasing age, leaving children unaffected and as susceptible as before, a hypothesis that became the principal rationale for mandatory revaccination in the 1990s.

Unfortunately, the concept of revaccination had already been abandoned, after a 1980 study demonstrated that previously vaccinated children with declining antibody titers responded minimally and for an unacceptably short time to booster doses of the measles vaccine.[5] Further refutation came from a sustained outbreak of 235 cases in Dane County, Wisconsin, over a nine-month period in 1986, of which the vast majority occurred among 5 to 19 year olds, only 6 percent of whom had not been vaccinated.[6]

To their surprise, the investigators of this outbreak found that "mild measles" (defined as typical rash with minimal fever) was far more prevalent in children who *lacked* vaccine-specific antibodies than it was in either unvaccinated children or those whose vaccinations had "taken" properly. This finding suggested that the vaccine virus was responsible for some inapparent or latent activity that had not been suspected before and did not show up on routine serological investigation.

Despite considerable evidence that the "immunity" conferred

by the measles vaccine might not be genuine, very few investigators have dared to consider such a possibility. Quite the contrary, the medical authorities have persuaded many state leg-
islatures to allocate additional funds for tighter enforcement
of existing vaccination laws. In some inner cities with high incidence, the vaccination age has been lowered to nine months,
recapitulating pre-1979 standards, when millions of children were
"inappropriately vaccinated" according to guidelines in force
since 1985. Now, as then, absurd vacillations and rigid assumptions are catching millions of innocent children in their web.

At present, the "final solution" to the measles question is
revaccination, with medical and public health authorities gen-
erously throwing in the mumps and rubella vaccines for good
measure. A bill currently before the Ohio legislature, for example, mandates documented proof of MMR (measles-mumps-
rubella) revaccination before a child can enter seventh grade.[7]
Once again, public compliance is being required with little
more justification than that the original dose was a failure and
the extra one cannot possibly hurt.

Other Vaccines

This generic faith continues to bless the pharmaceutical
industry in its endless and immensely profitable quest for new
vaccines, which in the present political climate is easily transformed into official authorization for vaccinating almost anyone against anything at any time.

In the late 1980s, a vaccine was introduced against *Hemophilus
influenza* type b, in response to scattered outbreaks of meningitis in crowded daycare facilities. At first purely optional for two

to four year olds, it soon became compulsory for all infants, including those not in daycare. The vaccine is presently given at or before 18 months of age, mostly along with the DPT before the child's first birthday.

Hepatitis B was primarily a disease of adult IV drug users, until it found its way into blood banks and became an institutionalized risk for people receiving transfusions and whole blood products. Developed in the 1970s, the hepatitis B vaccine is now being foisted on the entire population because medical authorities have never figured out how to effectively approach or target the drug subculture. In the past few months, the Centers for Disease Control (CDC) and the American Academy of Pediatrics have decided to mandate hepatitis B vaccination for all newborns.[8] Whether or not the American public, increasingly upset about vaccinations in general, will simply acquiese in this latest baptism of its newborn children remains to be seen.

The search goes on, inextricably linked to the technology of genetic engineering. The chicken pox vaccine, created in the 1970s but never successfully marketed, lacks only an official justification. Currently in the developmental stages are vaccines against Group A streptococcus as well as viruses associated with the common cold and bronchiolitis, all being bred into the gene pool of mice, rats, baboons, and other experimental animals, with no discernible caution or restraint.[9] Also on the horizon is an AIDS vaccine, monstrous even in principle because the people most in need of it are already seriously immunocompromised. A suppressive vaccine given to everyone would not only increase the odds of developing AIDS for those already at high risk; it would soften up the general population as well.

The DPT Story

The DPT (diphtheria-pertussis-tetanus) story remains the major battleground of the vaccine controversy in the United States. Thanks to consumer organizations such as Dissatisfied Parents Together (DPT), books such as Harris L. Coulter and Barbara Loe Fisher's *DPT: A Shot in the Dark*, and other grassroots initiatives at the political level, the plight of vaccine-injured children is coming to light.

In 1986, despite intensive lobbying by the American Medical Association (AMA) and other vested interest groups, Congress belatedly enacted the National Childhood Vaccine Injury Act, which requires the Public Health Service (PHS) to investigate all reports of vaccine injury and formulate guidelines for compensation.[10] Unfortunately, with a large part of its budget earmarked for advocating and enforcing compulsory vaccination programs, the PHS and its subsidiary agency, the CDC, can generally be counted on to look the other way. Indeed, the new DPT compensation guidelines rule out all conditions other than a few acute reactions (collapse, anaphylaxis, and brain damage) and the comparatively rare cases of chronic encephalopathy or brain damage appearing within seven days of vaccination.[11]

As the DPT battle continues, the unit cost of the vaccine is skyrocketing, as are the number and size of personal injury awards granted and personal injury claims filed against manufacturers. When parents insist, many pediatricians are now willing to give the DT vaccine alone.

Meanwhile, pertussis itself has made a slight comeback, with the CDC reporting a total of about 10,500 cases in the three-year interval from 1986 through 1988.[12] The demographics, however, remain effectively concealed behind bureaucratic terminology. Of those with "known vaccination status," 63 percent had been "inappropriately immunized," and 34 percent had not been vaccinated at all. Because very few cases appear to have occurred in the "appropriately vaccinated" group, the inference is that the vaccine is nearly 100 percent effective. Only by reading the fine print do we learn that those with "unknown vaccination status" (7,700 cases) comprised more than 70 percent of the total. And only by reading between the lines do we reach the patent conclusion that most, if not all, of the "unknown" group must have been vaccinees with no acceptable documentation.

Yet, at least in official circles, faith reigns supreme. One Philadelphia pediatrician, noting several cases of pertussis in infants less than two months of age, recently advocated that the DPT be given even earlier—"as early in life as possible."[13]

Vaccine-Related Illness

Whereas modern medicine seeks to define itself *quantitatively*, as a set of technologies for identifying and controlling key numbers, the task of the healer is essentially *qualitative*, to derive the treatment from the unique energy of each patient. As such, a large body of case material has emerged suggesting that vaccines tend to weaken the immune system of many individuals. In addition to immediate reactions (high fever, aberrant behavior, and others), chronic illness (asthma, eczema, allergies, recurrent otitis media, learning "disabilities," and more) has been linked to several of the vaccines.

This connection is confirmed in some cases by pathological evidence that the nosode, or homeopathic remedy derived from the vaccine itself, proves useful in treating the illness. In other instances, children are helped by many of the same remedies as would have been useful had they not been affected by the vaccine.[14] In other words, the vaccine connection cannot be proved but only suspected, suggesting that the vaccines often act *nonspecifically* to deepen a child's preexisting chronic disease tendency.

A complete picture of how the vaccines act inside the human body will require controlled scientific investigations into vaccinated and unvaccinated children over a period of many years, based on each child's total health picture over time. Only by making vaccines entirely optional, a status they have in many European countries, is this research possible. Society thus owes a considerable debt of gratitude to those parents who have decided not to vaccinate.

An Alternative Theology of Healing

Lest anyone supposes that religious concepts have no place in medicine, here are three aphorisms of the great 16th-century physician Paracelsus, offering a practical and ecumenical theology that healers of all disciplines can accept and live by without having to ram them down anybody's throat:

"The art of healing comes from Nature, not the physician."

"Every illness has its own remedy within itself."

"A man could not be born alive and healthy were there not already a physician hidden in him."[15]

Taken together, these sayings amount to a summary of most

everything the present medical system has left out, namely:

■ Healing implies wholeness. The verb to *heal* comes from the same Anglo-Saxon root as *whole*. Healing means simply to make whole again. Because it represents a concerted response of the entire organism, it implies a totality, a purely qualitative integration on a deeper level than can be defined by any assemblage of parts or approximated by any quantitative measurement.

■ All healing is self-healing. As a fundamental property of all living systems, healing is going on all the time and tends to complete itself spontaneously, with or without external assistance. This means that the role of physicians and other healers is essentially to assist and enhance the natural process that is already under way.

■ Healing applies only to individuals. Healing pertains to individuals in unique here-and-now situations rather than to abstract diseases, principles, or categories. In other words, it is an *art*, and can never be reduced to a technique or procedure, however scientific its foundation.

To these principles one could add a fourth, governing the doctor-patient relationship and subsisting as a fundamental political and legal right: *Health, illness, birth, and death are inalienable life experiences belonging wholly to the people undergoing them. Nobody else has the right to manipulate or control them, or any part of the body involved in them, without their explicit request or that of somebody authorized by them to act on their behalf.*

A fifth postulate, from the writings of Lao Tzu, would provide an appropriate bottom-line criterion:

A leader is best when people barely know he exists,

Not so good when people obey him and acclaim him,

Worst when they despise him.

Of a good leader, when his work is done and his aim is
fulfilled,

The people will say, "We did this ourselves."[16]

Notes

1. R. Mendelsohn, *Confessions of a Medical Heretic* (Chicago: Contemporary Books, 1979), pp. xiv et seq.

2. J. Cherry, "The New Epidemiology of Measles and Rubella," *Hospital Practice* (July 1980): 49; and L. Markowitz et al., "Patterns of Transmission in Measles Outbreaks in the U.S.," *New England Journal of Medicine 320,* no. 77 (12 January 1989).

3. B. Nkowane et al., *American Journal of Public Health 77* (1987): 434–438.

4. R. Chen et al., *American Journal of Epidemiology 129* (1989): 173–182.

5. See Note 2 (Cherry), p. 52.

6. M. Edmondson et al., "Mild Measles and Secondary Vaccine Failure during a Sustained Outbreak in a Highly Vaccinated Population," *Journal of the American Medical Association 263* (9 May 1990): 2467–2471.

7. LSC 119 0411-1, Sub. HB 168, Ohio General Assembly (1991–1992).

8. *Boston Globe* (11 June 1991): 1–F.

9. "Medical News and Perspectives," *Journal of the American Medical Association 262* (20 October 1989): 2055.

10. Vaccine Adverse Event Reporting System (VAERS), Public Health Service (1986).

11. Ibid., "Reportable Events Following Vaccination," table 1.

12. "Pertussis Surveillance: U.S., 1986–1988," *Journal of the American Medical Association 263* (23 February 1990): 1058–1069.

13. *Family Practice News* (15 November 1990): 6.

14. Documented case studies appearing in the original text will be published in a forthcoming issue of the *Journal of the American Institute of Homeopathy.*

15. P. A. T. B. von Hohenheim, *Selected Writings of Paracelsus,* J. Jacobi, ed., N. Guterman, trans. (New York: Pantheon, 1958), pp. 50, 76.

16. Lao Tzu, *The Way of Life,* W. Bynner, trans. (New York: Perigree Books, 1972), p. 6.

Adapted, with permission, from a lecture given by Richard Moskowitz, MD, at the Annual Conference of the Society of Homeopaths, in Manchester, UK, September 14, 1991.

HEPATITIS B VACCINE

Dear *Mothering,*

The Centers for Disease Control (CDC) has recommended a series of three vaccinations against hepatitis B for all infants and teenagers. Hepatitis B is considered a sexually transmitted disease, affecting especially those who share intravenous drug needles or who have multiple sexual partners. The vaccine will not be voluntary as are other preventive measures for sexual health, such as condom use. Moreover, most children will be vaccinated before reaching an age at which they can make decisions about drug use and sexual activity.

For *infants?* The "experts" say this is the best course to take to ensure that all young people are protected before they become sexually active. I say, "Enough is enough!" Not even exemptions are guaranteed: almost all states have a built-in provision to rescind exemptions in the case of an epidemic declared by health authorities.

The mandating of the hepatitis B vaccine is expected to be taken on in most 1992 legislative sessions, "at the request of the Department of Health." In some states, such as New Mexico, the vaccine will automatically become required because immunization law states that vaccines considered "standard medical practice" should be adopted by the state.

I urge readers to keep this vaccine from becoming law before it is too late. Stand up, and take action. Share the information. Write to your state legislators, and inform them that you do not want to see the hepatitis B vaccine mandated in 1992, or any other year, and make sure they know you are serious. The CDC recommendation is an inappropriate, unethical, and unacceptable way to handle the problem of hepatitis B infection.

Bonnie Plumeri Franz
Ogdensburg, New York

MORE ON VACCINATIONS

Dear *Mothering*,

Thank you for your article "Vaccination: A Sacrament of Modern Medicine" by Richard Moskowitz, MD (Spring 1992). My children's pediatrician tried to discourage me from eliminating the pertussis from their round of vaccines. I said, "No, thank you. I grew up with a younger sister who was among the 1 in 365,000 likely to experience a strong adverse reaction to the shot."

My sister is mentally and physically disabled, and battles seizures on a daily basis. In 1958, my father knew her condition was a reaction to the pertussis vaccine. He still remembers the high fever and the vomiting, and recalls vividly how his little daughter, who was "born perfect," cried endlessly the day of her shot. Not until the late 1960s did the mass media come out on the subject, with reports of lawsuits being filed against pharmaceutical companies. Media coverage continues today, although we are not told that the official statistics of risk reflect only "reported" reactions to the vaccine. The American Medical Association (AMA) has been using "cerebral palsy" as a catchall diagnosis to avoid acknowledging the real culprit, and the current trend is to include SIDS as an escape diagnosis.

Your informative articles support my suspicions about the pertussis and other unnecessary, if not harmful, vaccines. My parents would have been thankful for this information 32 years ago when vaccinations were the "thing to do." We would have gladly traded a shot for a lifetime of watching a loved one struggle from day to day.

I, like many others, await each action-packed issue of *Mothering*. The articles are strong and the subjects often controversial, leading me to new insights and challenges in my approach to mothering and helping me view other approaches with an open mind. Each issue inspires me to write and get involved, yet never so much as this one did.

Denise Shaffer
Rohnert Park, California

Dear Dr. Moskowitz,

When I first became a mother, I was afraid to look at some of the issues concerning my baby's health. Due to my ignorance and fear of "knowing too much" (a phrase used by one of my obstetricians), I allowed my daughter to be vaccinated several times. Then I sent away for *Mothering*'s booklet *Vaccinations*. After reading it and talking with mothers who had opted not to have their children vaccinated, I decided against further inoculations.

The last vaccination my daughter received was the MMR vaccine, at 16 months of age. Prior to that, she had three DPT shots, resulting in fever, lumps at the vaccination site, and personality changes lasting about three days. I, myself, have multiple allergies—which I now know is a contraindication for the DPT vaccine.

My daughter, three years old and still nursing, has demonstrated sensitivities to quite a few foods and environmental substances. She has had one ear infection (we try to avoid dairy products), which we treated with antibiotics. And she always seems to look "lousy." My question is: Now that the damage is done, is there any way to repair it? How does one go about rebuilding the immune system? Is there a way to expel the vaccines?

Every time I read about the dangers of vaccines, I want to cry. What's done is done, however. And as much as I would like to, I can't turn back the clock. Is there an answer?

Renee M. Farina
West Willington,
Connecticut

Dear Renee,

I can assure you that your daughter's condition is not uncommon or serious, and will undoubtedly heal itself in time even if nothing is done. The pro-

cess could very possibly be speeded up and made more efficient with the aid of homeopathy and other natural therapies as well as a qualified professional who is well skilled in these methods.

Richard Moskowitz, MD
Watertown,
Massachusetts

Dear Friends of *Mothering*,

Before the birth of our first child, my husband and I did a lot of research and decided not to allow our children to be vaccinated. In the 11 years since, we have continued to educate ourselves on the subject, keeping up on the latest vaccine trends and developments. Not once have we come across information that would lead us to question our decision. In fact, we are more adamantly opposed to vaccinations today than we were in the beginning.

We have two wonderfully

healthy sons who have never suffered the string of "common" illnesses that medical practitioners regard as normal to childhood. Indeed, I was shocked when a family practitioner recently told me that children today will have an average of three ear infections before their first birthday. This goes far beyond acceptable definitions of the term "epidemic," and yet it is considered normal, as is the implanting of ear tubes.

I am convinced that breastfeeding each of my babies for a full three years has played a major role in their overall good health. And I firmly believe that allowing their immune systems to develop naturally, free of artificially produced antigens, has left their bodies strong and vigorous.

With so much in the news about AIDS, I often wonder if there is a connection between this immune deficiency and the use of vaccines. I would be very interested to know if anyone has researched the effects of HIV on unvaccinated populations. Are individuals infected with HIV more likely to develop AIDS if they were fully vaccinated in their youth? Could it be that toying with the immune system through routine childhood vaccines leaves the system so weakened (or undeveloped) that it is unable to fight off this virus later in life?

For me and my family, far too many questions have not been asked, much less answered, to justify adherence to AMA vaccination guidelines. We have endured criticism for our decision—something far more bearable than the guilt we would suffer were we to vaccinate and find out later just how damaging this practice is. In our hearts, we know we have made the right choice.

Sarah Logan
Waco, Texas

Dear Editors,

We applaud Lynne McTaggart's "The MMR Vaccine" (Spring 1992). Your magazine's continual effort to question mandatory vaccination is deeply appreciated.

Parental choice in children's health care is a key issue. It should be the right of parents to choose the kind of care they believe is best for their children. Thank you for this reminder.

M. Victor Westberg, Manager
Committees on Publication
The First Church of
Christ, Scientist
Boston, Massachusetts

RESOURCES FOR FURTHER STUDY ON VACCINATIONS

Organizations

Alternatives in Mothering, Inc. (AIM)
629 Brick Blvd., Suite 439
Brick, NJ 08723
A nonprofit support group for families seeking information and resources on immunizations and alternative health choices. Send SASE for information and order form. Quarterly newsletter: $18.00 per year. Available reprints include *Immunization Information and Resource List*, $5.00.

Aurum Healing Centre.
PO Box 1198
Geelong 3220
Australia
052-29-7697
Isaac Golden
Publishes *Vaccination? A Review of Risks and Alternatives.* Includes a specific homeopathic program for protection from common childhood diseases as an alternative to vaccination, and a sup-

plementary homeopathic program if exposed to infection. A\$20 surface, A\$25 airmail as an Australian bank draft.

The Clymer Health Clinic
5724 Clymer Road
Quakertown, PA 18951
A set of three publications on vaccination, written in part by Dr. Harold E. Buttram, is available from the clinic: *The Dangers of Immunization, Vaccinations and Immune Malfunction,* and *How to Legally Avoid Unwanted Immunization.* \$12.00 per set postpaid.

Hahnemann Pharmacy
828 San Pablo
Albany, CA 94706
510-527-3003
This organization specializes in homeopathic remedies, many of which are made on the premises. *The Immunization Decision* by Randall Neustaedter is available directly from them for \$8.95 plus \$4.00 shipping/handling (if prepaid).

The Immunisation Awareness Society, Inc.
PO Box 56048
Dominion Road
Auckland
New Zealand
Formed in 1988 to ensure that all parents have sufficient information to enable them to make an informed choice about vaccination. The society believes that people can only give informed consent to this medical procedure if they have access to all the

information available, for and against vaccination. Newsletter subscriptions: NZ$15 to NZ$25 (sliding scale).

The National Center for Homeopathy
801 N. Fairfax St., Suite 306
Alexandria, VA 22314
703-548-7790
A booklet, *The Case against Immunizations* by Richard Moskowitz, MD, is available from them for $3.00 plus $1.50 shipping/handling. An excerpt from the booklet is included in this publication.

The National Health Federation
212 W. Foothill Blvd.
PO Box 688
Monrovia, CA 91016
818-357-2181
An immunization kit is available for $10.00 plus $2.50 shipping/handling. The kit includes reprints of the following: *Does Your State Exempt Immunizations?; Certificate of Exemption; How to Avoid Compulsory Immunizations; The Truth about Immunizations* by Robert Mendelsohn, MD; *Your Right to Refuse Immunizations; Measles: A Mother's Refusal; Dangers of Immunizations; Vaccines: Friend or Foe?*

National Vaccine Information Center
Dissatisfied Parents Together
204-F Mill St.
Vienna, VA 22180
703-938-DPT3
The National Vaccine Information Center, operated by Dissat-

isfied Parents Together, is a national nonprofit educational organization representing parents and healthcare professionals concerned about childhood diseases and vaccines. The center provides support to help educate parents about vaccine safety and their right to choose immunizations, as well as support for parents and families who have experienced the devastation of a vaccine reaction, injury, or death. The book *DPT: A Shot in the Dark* is available for $13.00 (VA residents add $.45 state tax) and a booklet, *Whooping Cough: The DPT Vaccine and Reducing Vaccine Reactions*, for a $5.00 donation. For a $20.00 membership donation you will receive newsletters and other numerous publications, free to members, on vaccine compensation, other resources, studies, federal compensation, lawyers handling vaccine issues, and conflict of interest involved in the vaccine controversy.

National Vaccine Injury Compensation Program
Health Resources and Services Administration
Parklawn Building, Room 7-90
5600 Fishers Lane
Rockville, MD 20857
800-338-2382
Administered by the Department of Health and Human Services to provide payments for persons who have died or suffered an injury associated with vaccines for DPT, measles, mumps, and rubella, as well as oral and inactivated polio vaccine.

Vaccination Alternatives
Promoting Informed Choice
PO Box 346

New York, NY 10023
212-870-5117
Director: Sharon Kimmelman
Vaccination Alternatives offers facts, provides supportive coun-
seling, and empowers the individual with the right of refusal.
With this information each person is encouraged to make their
own decision regarding their health choices for themselves
and their children. Introductory information $3 plus SASE.

Publications

Dangers of Compulsory Immunizations: How to Avoid Them Legally
by lawyer Tom Finn, PO Box 1658, New Port Richey, FL 34656.

The Doctor's People
1578 Sherman Ave., #314
Evanston, IL 60204
The Doctor's People newsletter is no longer being published, however back issues are available for $2.50 each, and Dr. Robert Mendel-
sohn's books can also be purchased from them.

DPT: A Shot in the Dark
Harris L. Coulter and Barbara Loe Fisher
Harcourt Brace Jovanovich
1985. $13.00
Available directly from the National Vaccine Information Cen-
ter, DPT, 204-F Mill St., Vienna, VA 22180. 703-938-DPT3.

Honor Publications
PO Box 346
Cutten, CA 95534
Ida Honorof publishes *Report to the Consumer*, a newsletter on health related topics that often scoops the major media. Subscription: $8.00 per year. She also hosts a consumer oriented radio show on KPFK in Southern California.

The Immunization Decision
Randall Neustaedter
North Atlantic Books; 1990
Homeopathic Education Services, Berkeley, California.

Immunization: The Reality behind the Myth
Walene James
Bergin & Garvey
670 Amherst Road
South Hadley, MA 01075
1988. $10.95

Institute for Vaccine Research
PO Box 4182
Northbrook, IL 60065
708-272-5887
Josephine Szczesny
Publishes a reference list of scientific articles citing adverse reactions to vaccinations. $3.00. Also, an immunization packet: *"Yes" or "No"* for $25.00.

Dr. Daniel Lander
Family Chiropractor
RR1, Box 1106
Coopers Mills, ME 04341
Dr. Daniel Lander's pamphlet *On Immunization* is available for $2.50 postpaid. An updated version of his 1980 book *Chiropractic and Wholistic Health* will be available directly from him in 1993.

New Atlantean Press
PO Box 9638-20
Santa Fe, NM 87504
New Atlantean Press publishes *Vaccines: Are They Really Safe and Effective?* : *A Parent's Guide to Childhood Shots* by Neil Z. Miller. The book evaluates "mandated" vaccines to determine their safety, effectiveness, long-term effects, and the true cause of a decline in each disease. 80 pages, 12 charts, more than 300 citations. The book is available for $9.50 postpaid.

Vaccination, Social Violence and Criminality: The Medical Assault on the American Brain. Harris L. Coulter, North Atlantic Books, 1990.

What Doctors Don't Tell You Newsletter
Lynne McTaggart
4 Wallace Road
London N1 2PG
England

Other books from *Mothering*

THE WAY BACK HOME *(essays on life and family)*

CIRCUMCISION

SCHOOLING AT HOME: PARENTS, KIDS, AND LEARNING

BEING A FATHER: FAMILY, WORK, AND SELF

MIDWIFERY AND THE LAW

TEENS: A FRESH LOOK

Write for a free catalog of current publications—

Mothering, PO Box 1690, Santa Fe, NM 87504